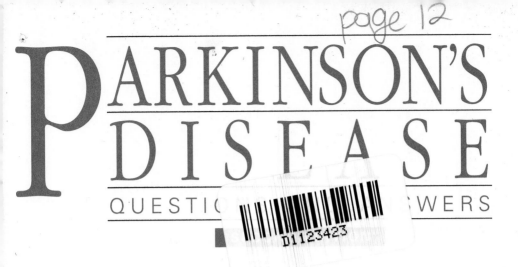

PARKINSON'S DISEASE

QUESTIONS AND ANSWERS

ROBERT A. HAUSER
Associate Professor of Neurology
Director, Parkinson's Disease and Movement Disorders Center
University of South Florida College of Medicine
Chief, Section of Neurology, Tampa General Hospital, Tampa, Florida

THERESA A. ZESIEWICZ
Assistant Professor of Neurology
Assistant Director, Parkinson's Disease and Movement Disorders Center
University of South Florida College of Medicine
Tampa General Hospital, Tampa, Florida

Foreword by
WILLIAM KOLLER
Professor and Chairman, Department of Neurology
University of Kansas Medical Center

merit
PUBLISHING
INTERNATIONAL

To our spouses and children,

for their love, support and encouragement.

merit

PUBLISHING
INTERNATIONAL

PARKINSON'S DISEASE
QUESTIONS AND ANSWERS

SECOND EDITION

MERIT PUBLISHING INTERNATIONAL

European address:
35 Winchester Street
Basingstoke
Hampshire RG21 7EE
England

North American address:
8260 NW 49th Manor
Pine Grove, Coral Springs
Florida 33067
U.S.A.

ISBN 1 873413 46 7

ROBERT A. HAUSER

THERESA A. ZESIEWICZ

merit
PUBLISHING
INTERNATIONAL

PARKINSON'S DISEASE

CONTENTS

FOREWORD

Parkinson's disease is a common disease of the nervous system. In the United States alone, this condition affects as many as one million people, although many patients go undiagnosed and others are not treated properly. Parkinson's disease is a complex affliction with both motor and non-motor symptomatology. Complications of long-term therapy can compromise treatment and tax the skill of even the most experienced clinician.

Parkinson's disease must be differentiated from other neurological conditions to make the proper diagnosis. The timing and selection of treatments require a thorough understanding of disease symptoms and both the benefits and side effects of medications and surgeries used to treat the disease. Physicians need to acquaint themselves with the promising new medical and surgical treatments now available.

The second edition of Parkinson's Disease-Questions and Answers by Robert Hauser and Theresa Zesiewicz poses important questions related to Parkinson's disease and discusses in an eloquent manner simple, practical and direct answers which clinicians require to diagnose and treat the disease. The publication is well illustrated, helping the reader to further understand the essential questions that are proposed. The answers to these important questions are direct and written in a manner that is easy to comprehend. Finally, the authors have succeeded in reducing very complex issues into practical management plans which summarize our expanding base of knowledge about Parkinson's disease

The book is divided into nine chapters. The first chapter discusses clinical features followed by the differential diagnosis of Parkinson's disease. A chapter on the causes of Parkinson's disease is next, followed by five chapters which look at therapy and medications available for the condition. Within these chapters is a comprehensive discussion of the complications associated with long term treatment, and other medical management issues are thoroughly examined and outlined. The last chapter in the book reviews the renewed interest in the surgical treatment of Parkinson's disease.

Any clinician involved with Parkinson's disease will benefit from this publication. Management is clearly discussed and the text gives firm ideas as to how to address the many problems associated with caring for patients with Parkinson's disease. The authors should be complimented on achieving a clear and thorough discussion of the management and treatment of Parkinson's disease.

William Koller, M.D., Ph.D.
Professor and Chairman
Department of Neurology
University of Kansas Medical Center

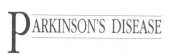

PARKINSON'S DISEASE

PARKINSON'S DISEASE

QUESTIONS AND ANSWERS

SECOND EDITION

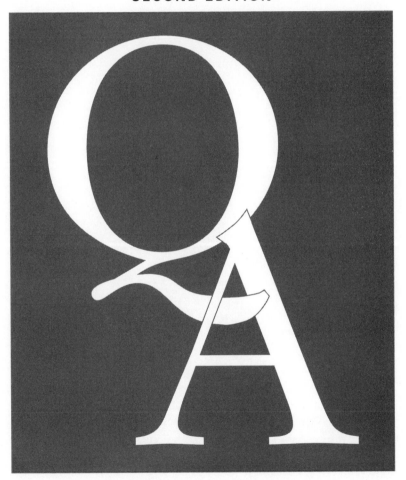

ROBERT A. HAUSER

THERESA A. ZESIEWICZ

merit

PUBLISHING
INTERNATIONAL

CHAPTER 1

INTRODUCTION TO PARKINSON'S DISEASE

Parkinson's disease is a progressive, neurologic disorder caused by a degeneration of dopaminergic neurons. James Parkinson first described the disease in 1817[1]. Since then, tremendous advances have been made in understanding its pathophysiology and in developing effective treatments. The landmark discovery that levodopa ameliorates symptoms came in the late 1960s. Even today, Parkinson's disease remains one of the few neurodegenerative diseases whose symptoms can be improved with medication therapy. Exciting research into emerging medical and surgical treatments continues at a breathtaking pace. This chapter introduces Parkinson's disease, its history, and current concepts of pathophysiology.

What causes the symptoms of Parkinson's disease?

Movement in the human body is produced by the motor cortex. The main motor pathway consists of the pyramidal system which extends from the motor cortex to the spinal cord. Lower motor neurons carry signals from the spinal cord to muscle to produce movement. The pyramidal system is modulated by the "extrapyramidal" circuit, which includes the substantia nigra, striatum, subthalamic nucleus, the external and internal segments of the globus pallidus, and the thalamus. The extrapyramidal system can either promote or inhibit movement depending on tonic dopamine innervation of the striatum. Normal movement is dependent on appropriate dopamine production by substantia nigra neurons innervating the striatum (figure 1-1).

Parkinson's disease is associated with a massive degeneration of dopaminergic nigrostriatal neurons. When approximately sixty to eighty percent of the dopamine producing neurons of the substantia nigra are lost, the extrapyramidal system is no longer able to effectively promote movement, and the symptoms of Parkinson's disease appear.

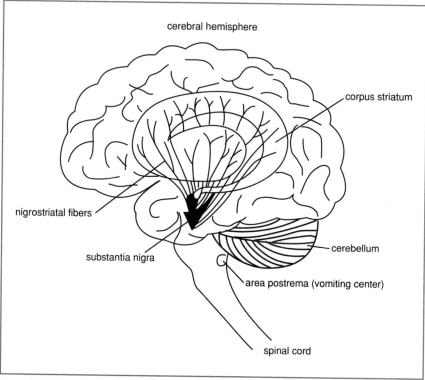

Figure 1-1. *Lateral view of the brain demonstrates dopamine neurons of the substantia nigra innervating the striatum.*

What are the clinical features of Parkinson's disease?

Parkinson's disease is clinically characterized by four main features:
- resting tremor (shaking back and forth when the limb is relaxed)
- bradykinesia (slowness of movement)
- rigidity (stiffness, or resistance of the limb to passive movement when the limb is relaxed)
- postural instability (poor balance).

Onset of symptoms is asymmetric with one limb, usually an arm, affected first. Signs and symptoms then spread to the other limb on that side and later affect the limbs of the opposite side. Resting tremor, bradykinesia, and rigidity are relatively early signs often apparent in the first-affected extremity. Postural instability is a late symptom typically emerging ten or more years into the disease. Other common signs include shuffling gait, stooped posture, difficulty with fine coordinated movements, and micrographia (small handwriting). Secondary features include autonomic dysfunction (constipation, sweating), cognitive symptoms (dementia), affective disturbances (depression), and sensory complaints including pain in muscles. These will be discussed in greater detail below.

How did Parkinson's disease get its name?

James Parkinson, a 19th century English physician, was the first to publish an accurate description of the disease in a pamphlet entitled, "An Essay on the Shaking Palsy"[1]. He had encountered several patients who exhibited resting tremor, stooped posture, shuffling gait, and retropulsion (falling backward). He recognized that symptoms progressively worsened, ultimately leading to death from complications due to immobility. The tremor was present with the limbs at rest. He dubbed the disease "paralysis agitans"; paralysis referring to the paucity of movement and agitans referring to the tremor. Although Parkinson did not identify abnormalities in muscle tone or cognition in his patients, the bulk of his description of the disease was remarkably accurate. The French physician Jean Marie Charcot added muscular rigidity, micrographia, sensory changes, and several other features to Parkinson's original description, and named it after the physician who first clearly described it[2].

Who gets Parkinson's disease?

Parkinson's disease commonly occurs in older individuals, although it may also occur in young adults. It is present worldwide and in all populations[3]. Although men have a slightly higher prevalence rate than women, the difference between sexes is small[4]. No race or specific region of the world has been found to be completely devoid of the disease.

What is the mean age of onset of Parkinson's disease?

The mean age of onset of Parkinson's disease is approximately 60 years. It usually occurs in patients over 50 years of age, and onset before age 25 is uncommon. The incidence and prevalence of the disease generally increase with increasing age[3]. Age-specific death rates for Parkinson's disease increased in the elderly in the United States from 1962 through 1984, and decreased in younger age groups[5]. The decreased mortality in younger individuals is likely the result of the introduction of dopamine replacement therapy.

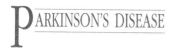

How common is Parkinson's disease?

"Prevalence" and "incidence" are two terms used to describe the frequency of a disease. Prevalence refers to the total number of people with the disease in a population at a given time. Incidence is the number of new cases of the disease diagnosed in a population during a given time period. Average crude prevalence rates for Parkinson's disease have been estimated at 120-180 per 100,000 in Caucasian populations[3] and the prevalence of the disease in individuals over 65 years of age is roughly 1%. Incidence rates have been estimated at 20 per 100,000. Studies conducted over the last century in Rochester, Minnesota have not uncovered a change in the prevalence of Parkinson's disease in the last fifty years[6].

Does Parkinson's disease occur more frequently in certain locations?

The highest prevalence of Parkinson's disease is in North America and Europe, while the lowest prevalence rates have been found in China, Japan, Nigeria, and Sardinia[3]. The Parsi community of Bombay, India was recently found to have the highest prevalence rates reported to date[7]. The Parsis are a people who migrated to India between the seventh and tenth centuries from Iran. They have a closed community, and rarely allow intermarriages with other races or religious groups. Whether genetic factors in a closed community or some environmental toxin present in the area is causing this high prevalence is unknown.

Is Parkinson's disease more common in Caucasians or African-Americans?

Studies conducted in the United States have generally found a lower prevalence of Parkinson's disease among African-Americans[8]. Even in Africa, the prevalence has been found to be lower in blacks than in whites or Indians[9]. However, in a door-to-door survey conducted in Copiah County, Mississippi prevalence among blacks was similar to that among whites when relatively loose diagnostic criteria were employed[10]. When more rigid diagnostic criteria were used, whites continued to have a higher prevalence. Further studies are needed to substantiate the belief that Parkinson's disease is more common in Caucasians.

What factors are associated with the development of Parkinson's disease?

There is interest in whether exposure to a toxin or multiple toxins might cause Parkinson's disease. It may not be coincidence that James Parkinson's original description of the disease in 1817 occurred at the beginning of the industrial revolution in the United States [11]. Several associations between environmental exposures and Parkinson's disease have been identified including rural living, well-water intake, vegetable farming, exposure to wood pulp, and exposure to pesticides [3]. Some of these associations are controversial and no environmental toxin has been identified that might be causative for most patients with Parkinson's disease. Nonetheless, interest in environmental toxins was greatly bolstered by the discovery that MPTP, a heroin derivative, caused a Parkinson's disease-like illness in young adults who injected themselves with this contaminant [12]. Animals which are made parkinsonian via injection of MPTP now provide a valuable research tool.

What is the prognosis of Parkinson's disease?

Parkinson's disease is a chronic, degenerative disease which usually progresses fairly slowly. Although an average rate of progression can be defined, it is not possible to accurately predict prognosis for an individual patient. Before the introduction of levodopa, Parkinson's disease dramatically reduced life expectancy. The mortality rate for Parkinson's disease patients was almost three times that of the general population. Treatment with dopamine replacement therapy essentially normalized life expectancy and death rates for Parkinson's disease and non-Parkinson's individuals are now approximately equal [13]. Most patients initially do very well on medication for four to six years. Between five and eight years most patients experience medication-related difficulty, and many develop poor balance by ten to twelve years. It takes an average of two and a half years to progress from stage to stage (see chapter 2), although this is only a rough guideline [13].

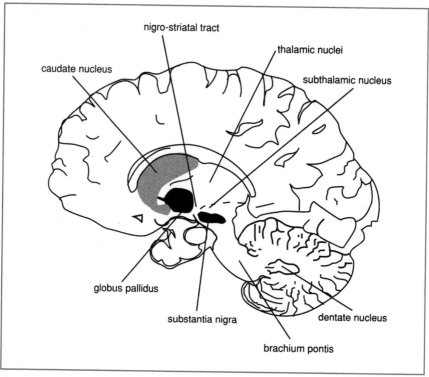

nigro-striatal tract

thalamic nuclei

caudate nucleus

subthalamic nucleus

globus pallidus

substantia nigra

dentate nucleus

brachium pontis

Figure 1-2. *Lateral view of the brain indicating positions of the substantia nigra, caudate, subthalamic nucleus and thalamus.*

What is the basic anatomy and pharmacology of Parkinson's disease?

The major symptoms of Parkinson's disease are due to abnormalities in the extrapyramidal motor circuit. The basal ganglia are subcortical nuclei comprised of three components: the caudate nucleus, the putamen and the globus pallidus (figure 1-2). The caudate nucleus consists of a "head" which lies next to the lateral ventricle, the "body" which lies lateral to the thalamus, and the "tail" which enters the temporal lobe. The putamen and globus pallidus lie between the internal and external capsules, with the putamen situated laterally. The globus pallidus is composed of medial and lateral segments. Also involved in the extrapyramidal circuit is the substantia nigra. This structure is located in the midbrain, ventral to the tegmentum. It is composed of a pigment-rich area called the "zona compacta" and a relatively cell-poor region called the "zona reticulata". Neurons in the zona compacta are responsible for the production of dopamine, while the zona reticulata primarily produces GABA (gamma-amino-butyric acid).

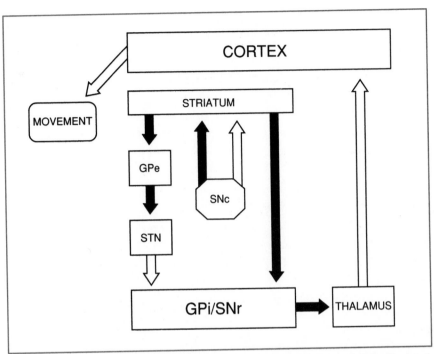

Figure 1-3. *Schematic representation of the normal motor circuit demonstrating the direct and indirect pathways. See text for details. Black arrows represent inhibition and white arrows represent stimulation. SNc = substantia nigra pars compacta; GPe = globus pallidus externa; STN = subthalamic nucleus; GPi = globus pallidus interna; SNr = substantia nigra pars reticulata.*

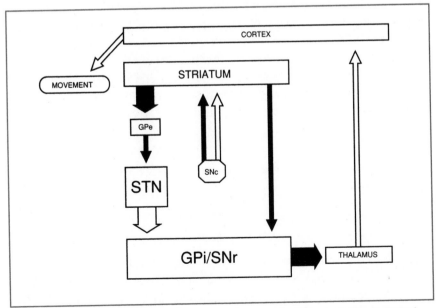

Figure 1-4. *Schematic representation of the motor circuit in Parkinson's disease. Decreased dopamine production by the SNc leads to overinhibition of the thalamocortical pathway. See text for details.*

The ability to produce movement is dependent on a complex motor circuit involving the substantia nigra, basal ganglia, subthalamic nucleus, thalamus, and the cerebral cortex (figure 1-3). Signals from the cerebral cortex are processed through the motor circuit and returned to the same areas by a feedback pathway [14]. The output from the motor circuit is directed through the internal segment of the globus pallidus (GPi) and the substantia nigra pars reticulata (SNr). This inhibitory output is directed to the thalamocortical pathway and suppresses movement. There are two pathways within the extrapyramidal system: a direct and an indirect pathway. In the direct pathway, outflow from the striatum (putamen and caudate) inhibits the GPi and SNr. The indirect pathway contains inhibitory connections between 1) the striatum and the external segment of the globus pallidus (GPe), and 2) the globus pallidus externa (GPe) and the subthalamic nucleus (STN). The subthalamic nucleus has an excitatory influence on the GPi and SNr. The GPi/SNr sends inhibitory efferents to the ventral lateral (VL) nucleus of the thalamus. Putamenal neurons containing D1 receptors comprise the direct pathway and project to the GPi. Putamenal neurons containing D2 receptors are part of the indirect pathway and project to the GPe. Dopamine activates the direct pathway, and inhibits the indirect pathway.

In Parkinson's disease, decreased production of dopamine by the SNc leads to increased inhibitory output from the GPi/SNr (figure 1-4). This increased inhibition of the thalamocortical pathway suppresses movement. Via the direct pathway, lowered dopamine levels decrease inhibition of the GPi/SNr, causing overinhibition of the thalamus. Via the indirect pathway, lowered dopamine levels increase inhibition of the GPe, resulting in "disinhibition" of the STN. Increased STN output promotes GPi/SNr inhibition of the thalamus.

What histopathologic features are associated with Parkinson's disease?

Parkinson's disease involves a degeneration of cells in the substantia nigra pars compacta substantia nigra. The lightly melanized ventral layer in the pars compacta is primarily affected [15]. Clinical manifestations occur when roughly sixty percent of neurons in this region are lost. Cell loss is not confined solely to the substantia nigra but also affects the locus ceruleus, thalamus, cerebral cortex, and autonomic nervous system. Neurotransmitter abnormalities involve the cathecholaminergic and serotonergic systems as well as the dopaminergic system.

The pathological determination of Parkinson's disease includes the identification of Lewy bodies [15]. These are eosinophilic, concentric, hyaline inclusions present in the cytoplasm of some remaining substantia nigra pars compacta neurons. They can also be found in the locus ceruleus, autonomic system, and other areas. Lewy bodies consist of a dense center composed of amorphous material and a pale staining, peripheral halo. The outer layer consists of cytoskeletal elements. The reason for their formation in Parkinson's disease is unknown but they may be a consequence of neuronal injury. Lewy bodies have been found in other degenerative disorders and in some elderly individuals without parkinsonian features. The presence of Lewy bodies at autopsy in some "normal" individuals may suggest that they had preclinical Parkinson's disease, and would have developed signs and symptoms if they had lived longer.

What is the neurochemistry of Parkinson's disease?

Dopamine and other cathecholamines are synthesized from tyrosine by the following pathway:

tyrosine ——> 3,4-dihydroxyphenylalanine (DOPA) ——> dopamine ——> norepinephrine ——> epinephrine.

The rate-limiting step in the formation of dopamine is the hydroxylation of tyrosine to form DOPA. This step is catalyzed by the protein tyrosine hydroxylase (figure 1-5).

Tyrosine hydroxylase is a marker of dopamine neurons. It is decreased in the substantia nigra of Parkinson's disease patients. Dopamine and its metabolites, homovanillic acid (HVA) and dihydroxyphenylacetic acid (DOPAC), are reduced in the striatum, the primary target of dopaminergic neurons [16]. Dopamine loss is more extensive in the putamen than in the caudate [17]. Dopamine levels are also reduced in the hypothalamus, mesolimbic, and mesocortical areas.

Once formed, dopamine is metabolized by two enzymes: monoamine oxidase (MAO), which deaminates dopamine intraneuronally, and catechol-O-methyl transferase (COMT), which methylates dopamine outside the neuron [18] (figure 1-6). MAO exists in two forms: MAO-A and MAO-B. MAO-B is the predominant form in the brain and is found on the outer membrane of mitochondria. MAO-B inhibitors increase levels of striatal dopamine. COMT methylates dopamine extraneuronally by

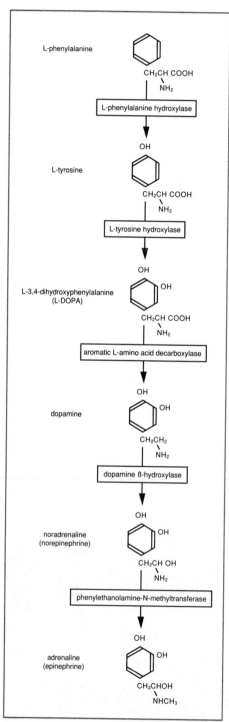

catalyzing the transfer of a methyl group from S-adenosyl-L-methionine to the m-hydroxy group of dopamine. Dopamine is also deactivated by neuronal reuptake via the dopamine transporter.

What are the different types of dopamine receptors?

Receptors are macromolecules composed of proteins which are located on neuronal membranes (figure 1-7). The two main type of dopamine receptors are D1 and D2 [19,20]. Dopamine functions by modulating the direct and indirect pathways of the extrapyramidal motor circuit through its effect on D1 and D2 receptors. Dopamine receptors are linked to a guanine nucleotide-binding protein (G-protein), to form a complex which interacts with adenyl cyclase to control formation of the second messenger, adenylate cyclase (figure 1-8). The D1 receptor family includes D1 and D5 receptors, while D2 includes D2, D3, and D4 (figure 1-9). Receptors in the D1 family increase cyclic AMP, while those in the D2 family reduce cyclic AMP [19-21]. D2 receptor activation is important in the anti-parkinsonian response to dopamine agonist medications. The role of D1 receptor activation in the response to medications is less clear.

Figure 1-5. *Synthesis of dopamine and other catecholamines.*

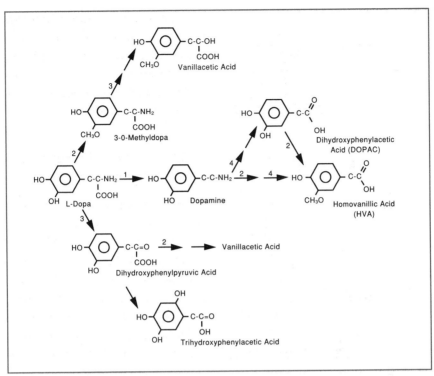

Figure 1-6. *Metabolism of levodopa and dopamine. 1=aromatic amino acid decarboxylase; 2=catechol-O-methyltransferase; 3=tyrosine aminotransferase; 4=monoamine oxidase.*

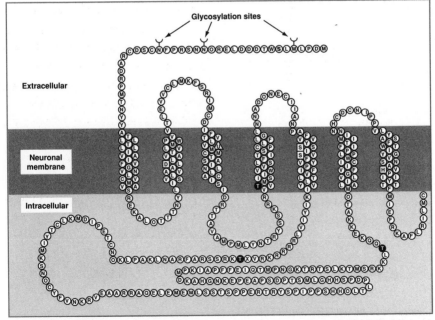

Figure 1-7. *Structure of D2 receptor. Each circle represents an amino acid. Black circles represent phosphorylation sites.*

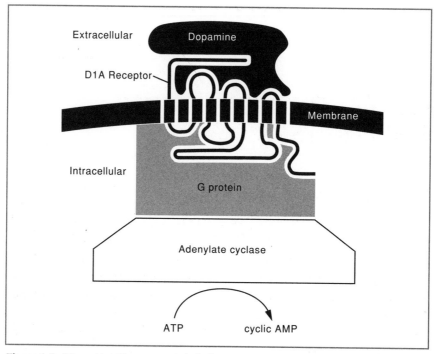

Figure 1-8. *D1 receptor. The receptor is linked to a G protein to control the synthesis of the second messsenger, cyclic AMP.*

Are there tests available to diagnose Parkinson's disease?

The diagnosis of Parkinson's disease is made by clinical evaluation and there are currently no simple, widely available laboratory tests which make the diagnosis. Fluorodopa positron emission tomography (PET) is a useful index of striatal dopaminergic function [22] but is expensive and not widely available. Single photon emission computerized tomography (SPECT) using radioisotopes that bind to the dopamine transporter on nigrostriatal neuron terminals is just emerging as a useful modality [23]. Further development of SPECT technology may provide a widely available and relatively inexpensive diagnostic tool for the near future.

	D1		D2		
Currently used term	A	B	A	B	C
Previously used term	D1	D5	D2	D3	D4
Location (high concentrations)	Striatum Nucleus accumbens Amygdala Olfactory bulb	Hippocampus Hypothalamus	Striatum Nucleus accumbens Substantia nigra Olfactory bulb	Hypothalamus Nucleus accumbens Olfactory bulb	Frontal cortex Midbrain Medulla
Action (information is limited to biochemical indexes)	Increases cyclic AMP	Increases cyclic AMP	Reduces cyclic AMP Opens potassium channels Closes calcium channels	Reduces cyclic AMP	Reduces cyclic AMP

Figure 1-9. *Distribution and function of dopamine receptors.*

CHAPTER 2

CLINICAL FEATURES OF PARKINSON'S DISEASE

What are the cardinal features of Parkinson's disease?

The four cardinal signs of Parkinson's disease are resting tremor, rigidity, bradykinesia, and postural instability. Tremor is the oscillation of a body part about a joint and is most commonly observed as "shaking back and forth." Rigidity refers to increased resistance when a joint is passively flexed and extended. Bradykinesia means slowness of movement. Postural instability refers to lack of balance and in contrast to the first three cardinal features does not emerge until late in the disease. The most common initial finding is an asymmetric resting tremor although about twenty percent of patients first experience clumsiness of a hand[1].

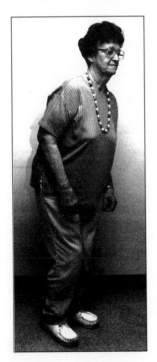

Figure 2-1. *Characteristic flexed posture of a patient with Parkinson's disease. (used with permission)*

What other clinical features are associated with Parkinson's disease?

Patients with early Parkinson's disease often notice difficulty with fine coordinated movements. Daily tasks may be more difficult to perform. There may be more difficulty buttoning shirts, combing one's hair or playing golf. Family members may notice a flattened facial expression (masked facies). The voice may become soft (hypophonia) and monotonal. The first-affected arm may not swing fully when walking, and the foot on the same side may scuff the floor. Axial posture becomes progressively flexed and strides are shortened (figure 2-1). Handwriting may be small and cramped (micrographia). The patient may eventually notice drooling and have difficulty swallowing foods. Pain may occur in an

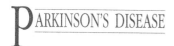

affected limb, leading to an erroneous diagnosis of arthritis or bursitis. Often this aching pain involves a large muscle group on one side of the body. Patients may complain of a change in the taste of food which is caused by a lack of smell (anosmia). Depression or dementia may emerge. Symptoms of autonomic dysfunction are common, including constipation, urinary frequency, sweating abnormalities, dermatitis, and sexual dysfunction. Patients may also experience sleep disturbances.

How does one make the diagnosis of Parkinson's disease?

The best clinical predictors of a pathology diagnosis of Parkinson's disease are:

◆ asymmetry of onset
◆ presence of resting tremor
◆ good response to levodopa therapy.

The clinical diagnosis of Parkinson's disease is made by evaluation of the patient's history, neurologic examination, and response to dopamine replacement therapy. There are no blood tests that make the diagnosis and brain CT and MRI are typically unrevealing.

The following categories have been proposed for a clinical diagnosis of idiopathic Parkinson's disease [2]:

◆ It is POSSIBLE that the patient has Parkinson's disease if one of the following is present: tremor (either resting or postural), rigidity, or bradykinesia.

◆ It is PROBABLE that the patient has Parkinson's disease if two of the major features (resting tremor, rigidity, bradykinesia, or postural instability) are present, or if resting tremor, rigidity, or bradykinesia are asymmetric.

◆ It is DEFINITE that the patient has Parkinson's disease if three of the major features are present, or if two of the features are present with one of them presenting asymmetrically.

Causes of secondary parkinsonism must be ruled out before a diagnosis of idiopathic Parkinson's disease can be made (see chapter 3). These include medications, cerebrovascular disease, toxins, infection, other degenerative disorders (Creutzfeld-Jacob disease, Gerstmann-Straussler, Wilson's disease, Huntington's disease, neuroacanthocytosis), normal pressure hydrocephalus, and metabolic abnormalities.

What are the clinical characteristics of the tremor of Parkinson's disease?

Resting tremor is the most common presenting feature of Parkinson's disease, affecting almost seventy percent of patients[1]. It may be present in one or more limbs and is often asymmetric. Tremor is typically present when the limb is at rest, but may also be seen with the limb in a position of postural maintenance (e.g., with the arms outstretched). The characteristic tremor is a "pill-rolling" movement of the fingers with a frequency of four to five cycles per second. The amplitude is quite variable and may change from minute to minute. The amplitude commonly increases in periods of stress such as when the patient is asked to perform a cognitive task. Like most tremors, it disappears during sleep. The resting tremor of Parkinson's disease can be the most difficult sign to treat because of its variable response to medication therapy.

What is akinesia and how does it differ from akathisia?

Akinesia means "lack of movement". It refers to slowness in the initiation and execution of movement experienced by Parkinson's disease patients. Parkinson's disease patients have longer reaction times coupled with an element of inattention which adds to their "slowness". This paucity of movement is often described as the most disabling feature of the disease.

Akathisia refers to a compulsion to move about and is commonly expressed as an inability to remain seated[3]. It may be seen in idiopathic Parkinson's disease, as well as post-encephalitic parkinsonism. The initial stages of akathisia involve an inner feeling of restlessness, followed by the need to move. Unlike levodopa-induced dyskinesia which is comprised of involuntary choreiform (random twisting, turning) movements, akathisia does not involve abnormal types of movement but rather an increased quantity of normal movements. Patients may march in place, pace back and forth, or exhibit repetitive movements of the limbs. Its exact etiology is unknown but probably related to insufficient dopamine innervation. In psychiatric patients, akathisia is commonly induced by anti-psychotic medications. In this setting, akathisia may be difficult to differentiate from the restlessness of psychotic agitation. Treatment of akathisia involves reduction of anti-dopaminergic medication, or the possible use of anticholinergics, antihistamines, or dopaminergic medications. Some studies have found beta-blockers to be helpful[3].

How do young and old onset Parkinson's disease patients differ?

From five to ten percent of Parkinson's disease patients experience symptoms before age forty[4]. A young patient who presents with parkinsonian features warrants a careful screen to rule out secondary causes of parkinsonism, especially those which are potentially treatable, such as Wilson's disease. Young onset Parkinson's disease patients are usually quite responsive to dopamine replacement therapy, have less dementia, and more readily experience levodopa-induced dyskinesias than their older counterparts[5]. Older patients are more likely to develop progressive bradykinesia that responds only partially to levodopa, and more likely to develop dementia.

How common is dementia in Parkinson's disease?

Dementia is defined as a loss of intellectual abilities of sufficient severity to interfere with social or occupational functioning[6]. The loss of intellectual function almost always involves memory impairment, and may be associated with personality changes, impaired judgment, and difficulty with abstract thinking. Dementia is fairly common in Parkinson's disease. Reported prevalence rates range from 10% to 80%[7], but actual rates are probably closer to 15% to 30%[8].

The "subcortical" dementia of Parkinson's disease differs from the "cortical" dementia of Alzheimer's disease. Subcortical dementia involves psychomotor retardation, memory difficulties, cognitive abnormalities, and mood alterations[9]. These features are thought to be caused by abnormalities in deep gray matter structures. Short-term memory may be specifically affected in patients with Parkinson's disease, while immediate recall and long-term memory remain fairly intact[10]. Patients with the dementia of Parkinson's disease may suffer with "bradyphrenia", or psychomotor slowing. They have increased processing times with longer response latencies. Visuospatial function may also be impaired. Dementia in Parkinson's disease may result from abnormalities in multiple neurotransmitter systems, including acetylcholine, norepinephrine, serotonin, dopamine, and somatostatin [10].

In contrast to subcortical dementia, cortical dementia commonly leads to aphasia, anomia, agnosia, and apraxia. Although Parkinson's disease patients are usually not aphasic, they may have difficulty with verbal fluency and with phrase construction.

How common is depression in Parkinson's disease patients?

Depression is the most commonly encountered "psychiatric" symptom in Parkinson's disease. As many as 40 to 50% of patients are affected by mood changes [11]. Depression in Parkinson's disease is more commonly associated with dysphoria and sadness, rather than self-blame or guilt [12]. It can occur at any time during the course of the disease and may emerge prior to motor symptoms. Several studies have reported a greater incidence of depression in female patients, but this remains controversial.

Depression in Parkinson's disease probably has both endogenous and reactive components. Several studies have found depressed patients to have lower levels of CSF 5-HIAA, the major metabolite of serotonin, as occurs in non-parkinsonian patients diagnosed with major depression [12]. Antidepressants are quite effective in treating depression associated with Parkinson's disease. Electroconvulsive therapy is considered for depressed patients who are refractory to medication.

Describe some of the autonomic disturbances associated with Parkinson's disease.

Autonomic dysfunction is an important cause of secondary features of Parkinson's disease.

James Parkinson described some of these characteristics in his original essay. Autonomic abnormalities may include the following:

- ◆ orthostatic hypotension
- ◆ dizziness
- ◆ constipation
- ◆ gastrointestinal disorders (decreased gastric emptying, swallowing difficulties)

- ◆ decreased salivation
- ◆ impotence
- ◆ sphincter dysfunction
- ◆ increased sweating
- ◆ heat intolerance
- ◆ seborrhea
- ◆ livedo reticularis.

As many as 70 to 80% of Parkinson's disease patients experience some degree of autonomic dysfunction [13]. Many patients develop a loss of variation in heart rate interval (R-R) in response to postural changes [14]. This is indicative of parasympathetic system dysfunction. Lewy bodies have been found in the lateral hypothalamus in Parkinson's disease patients, an area important to regulation of the parasympathetic system [15]. Autonomic dysfunction may also be caused by abnormalities in the sympathetic ganglia. Treatment of autonomic dysfunction is symptomatic.

Describe the sleep abnormalities of Parkinson's disease.

A common complaint of Parkinson's disease patients is the inability to get a full night of restful sleep. Patients describe both an inability to fall asleep and numerous nighttime awakenings. Patients may have difficulty falling asleep due to depression or persistent tremor. Early awakenings may be caused by a reemergence of symptoms at night as daytime medications wear off. Reemergence of tremor may turn a light arousal into a complete awakening. Rigidity and akinesia may make it impossible to turn over in bed. Some patients develop a reversal of sleep-wake patterns and may nap excessively during the day and remain awake at night. Sleep difficulties may also be caused by abnormalities in arousal mechanisms due to autonomic nervous system dysfunction [16]. In addition, endogenous levels of serotonin, important for slow wave sleep, are decreased in Parkinson's disease [17]. Patients may benefit from the judicious use of sleeping medications.

What are the stages of Parkinson's disease?

One way to describe the severity of Parkinson's disease is the Hoehn and Yahr scale, developed by Margaret Hoehn and Melvin Yahr in the 1960s [4]. This scale describes five "stages" of Parkinson's disease.

Stage I: Unilateral features of Parkinson's disease, including the major features of tremor, rigidity, or bradykinesia.

Stage II: Bilateral features mentioned above, along with possible speech abnormalities, decreased posture, and abnormal gait.

Stage III: Worsening bilateral features of Parkinson's disease, along with balance difficulties. Patients are still able to function independently.

Stage IV: Patients are unable to live alone independently.

Stage V: Patients need wheelchair assistance, or are unable to get out of bed.

The most commonly employed research scale is the Unified Parkinson's Disease Rating Scale (UPDRS). Individual features are graded on a 0 to 4 scale. These can be summed to arrive at subset scores for mentation, activities of daily living, and motor function, as well as a total score [18].

PARKINSON'S DISEASE

———

———

———

———

———

———

———

———

———

———

———

———

———

———

———

CHAPTER 3

DIFFERENTIAL DIAGNOSIS OF PARKINSON'S DISEASE

The differential diagnosis of Parkinson's disease is vast. Causes of secondary Parkinsonism include medications and toxins, cerebrovascular disease, infection, trauma, metabolic abnormalities, and brain neoplasms (figure 3-1). The "atypical parkinsonisms" are a group of degenerative disorders with clinical features that include bradykinesia and rigidity, but differ from Parkinson's disease both pathologically and clinically. The atypical parkinsonisms are characterized clinically by early speech and balance difficulty, with little or no response to dopaminergic therapy. This group of diseases includes progressive supranuclear palsy, corticobasal degeneration, and the multiple-system atrophies. The multiple system atrophies are marked clinically by a combination of extrapyramidal, pyramidal, autonomic and cerebellar abnormalities. Included in the multiple system atrophies are striatonigral degeneration, olivopontocerebellar atrophy, and Shy-Drager syndrome. This chapter will examine the differential diagnosis of Parkinson's disease, including characteristic features used to help recognize various diseases and possible therapies.

When should I be most suspicious that I am dealing with something other than Parkinson's disease?

One should always consider the differential diagnosis of Parkinson's disease before making a diagnosis. In all cases it is important to exclude the possibility of medication-induced parkinsonism. When dealing with young patients one's index of suspicion for other disorders should especially high as Parkinson's disease is generally a disease of older individuals. In patients with bradykinesia and rigidity, the combination of the absence of tremor and an inadequate response to dopaminergic medications greatly increases the likelihood that the correct diagnosis is not Parkinson's disease.

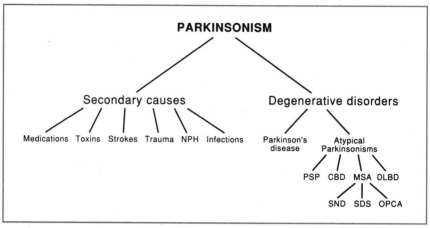

Figure 3-1. *The differential diagnosis of Parkinsonism.*
NPH=Normal Pressure Hydrocephalus   *CBD=Corticobasal Degeneration*
SND=Striatonigral Degeneration   *OPCA=Olivopontocerebellar Atrophy*
PSP=Progressive Supranuclear Palsy   *MSA=Multiple System Atrophy*
SDS=Shy-Drager Syndrome   *DLBD=Diffuse Lewy Body Disease*

Which medications cause parkinsonism?

Many pharmacologic agents can produce features of parkinsonism, including tremor, bradykinesia, rigidity, speech disturbances, and akathisia. These include dopamine-blockers such as the neuroleptics and antiemetics, as well as dopamine depletors such as reserpine and tetrabenazine. The gastrointestinal motility drug metochlopramide has both peripheral and central dopamine antagonism, and is probably the most underrecognized cause of medication induced parkinsonism today. Other drugs which may cause extrapyramidal signs include lithium[1], alpha-methyl-dopa[2], and some of the tricyclic antidepressants[3]. Antiepileptic medications may induce cerebellar symptoms[4] and valproic acid may cause tremor[5]. Patients presenting with parkinsonism who have recently taken any of these medications should be observed for at least six months off the medication before a diagnosis of Parkinson's disease is made[6].

Which toxins cause parkinsonism?

Toxins known to cause extrapyramidal symptoms include manganese, carbon monoxide, methanol, ethanol, and MPTP or 1-methyl-4-phenyl-1,2,3,6-tetrahydropyridine, a synthetic heroin derivative[7].

Which neurologic conditions mimic Parkinson's disease?

ARTERIOSCLEROTIC PARKINSONISM was first described by Critchley in the 1920's. "Vascular parkinsonism" is usually characterized clinically by akinesia and rigidity without tremor, and there may be other neurologic evidence of stroke [8]. Patients with multiple strokes may experience a step-wise progression of symptoms. An MRI should confirm the presence of cerebrovascular disease, although precise MRI criteria for a diagnosis of vascular parkinsonism are lacking. Tremor caused by cerebrovascular disease is uncommon, although there have been reports of unilateral tremor caused by vascular lesions in the thalamus [9]. Dystonia may be caused by strokes involving the basal ganglia.

INFECTIONS, including viruses such as HIV, and tuberculosis can cause extrapyramidal features. Postencephalitic parkinsonism is an historic example of an infectious cause of parkinsonism. "Encephalitis lethargica" or "von Economo's disease" occurred as an epidemic from 1919-1926. It commonly affected young adults in their 20s and 30s, but also involved a substantial number of children [10]. Early symptoms included fever, mental changes, and neurologic deficits consistent with encephalitis. Mortality rates were high. Those who survived were left with various neurologic deficits in the chronic encephalitic phase. Post-encephalitic parkinsonism developed weeks to years after the acute phase [11]. Parkinsonism was marked by bradykinesia and rigidity. Characteristic features included oculogyric crises with involuntary upward deviation of both eyes, and sleep rhythm disturbances. The parkinsonian features were often fairly stable and limited in progression. Pathologic changes were seen in the substantia nigra, subthalamic nucleus, and hypothalamus [10]. Very few post-encephalitic parkinsonism patients are alive today owing to the more than seventy years that have elapsed since the outbreak of encephalitis lethargica.

TRAUMA can also cause parkinsonism. Boxers who endure repeated trauma to the head may develop a syndrome of dementia, parkinsonism, pyramidal, and cerebellar signs [12]. "Dementia pugulistica" refers to the cognitive changes boxers experience years after the trauma occurred. Multiple concussions may cause diffuse axonal injury secondary to acceleration-deceleration forces affecting the brain. It is postulated that repeated head trauma may initiate dopamine neuronal degeneration.

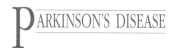

Pathologically, there is a loss of pigmented neurons in the substantia nigra, in the absence of Lewy bodies. Neurofibrillary tangles without senile plaques are found in the cerebral cortex[13].

NORMAL PRESSURE HYDROCEPHALUS is an acquired condition leading to changes in mentation, gait disturbances, and urinary incontinence. Patients develop overt bradykinesia without tremor. Gait apraxia mimics the shuffling gait of Parkinson's disease. The diagnosis is made by a combination of clinical and imaging findings. MRI should demonstrate hydrocephalus with the lateral ventricles dilated out of proportion to the cortical sulci and Sylvian fissures. Radionuclide cisternagram may demonstrate slow clearance of CSF. Some, but not all, patients will respond to shunting. Unfortunately, it is not currently possible to predict which patients will respond.

TUMORS and other mass lesions may occasionally lead to parkinsonian features. This can be caused by direct compression of the nigrostriatal tract by tumor or by stretching due to hydrocephalus.

What neurologic diseases are in the differential diagnosis of Parkinson's disease?

ESSENTIAL TREMOR (familial tremor) is marked by a postural tremor of the upper extremities not caused by a pharmacologic agent[14]. The disease usually occurs in patients who are over the age of forty and transmission is autosomal dominant although patients may lack a family history of tremor. The tremor is predominantly postural, often with a kinetic component. The postural component is observed with the arms outstretched and the kinetic component with the arms in motion such as when performing the finger-to-nose test. Its frequency is higher than that of Parkinson's disease, with a range of 4 to 12 Hz[15]. Essential tremor usually involves the upper extremities, is relatively symmetric, and is best seen with the arms outstretched, resulting in a flexion-extension or pronation-supination movement of the hands. The tremor slowly worsens over time[16]. Stressful activities may increase the amplitude, and ingestion of alcohol may temporarily relieve it. The arms are usually affected, while the legs and trunk are normally spared. Essential tremor commonly includes a head or voice tremor, whereas tongue, jaw, and lip tremors are more characteristic of Parkinson's disease. Other clinical manifestations of Parkinson's disease such as bradykinesia and rigidity are not present in essential tremor. Fifty to eighty percent of patients diagnosed with essential tremor will experience a good clinical response to propranolol or primidone [17]. However, this response is somewhat non-specific as the tremor of Parkinson's disease may also respond to these medications.

Essential tremor is often mistaken for Parkinson's disease. Essential tremor can be relatively asymmetric and can sometimes be seen with the arms in a position of rest. For this reason we do not make a diagnosis of Parkinson's disease in a patient who only has tremor, although a classic parkinsonian rest tremor does suggest the possibility that other cardinal features will develop over time. A five year history of bilateral upper extremity tremor without the emergence of bradykinesia or rigidity suggests a diagnosis of essential tremor rather than Parkinson's disease.

WILSON'S DISEASE is a disorder of copper metabolism transmitted by autosomal recessive inheritance [18]. The responsible gene has been mapped to the long arm of chromosome 13. Wilson's disease is a disease of children, adolescents and young adults. Symptoms rarely occur before age 6 or after age 40. In children, hepatobiliary symptoms predominate whereas in adolescents and young adults neuropsychiatric symptoms are the rule. The exact etiology is unknown but results in a positive copper balance. Free copper deposits in the liver and brain, leading to cirrhosis and neuropsychiatric features. The disease is associated with low levels of ceruloplasmin, a serum protein responsible for binding copper, increased liver copper concentration, and increased urinary copper excretion. Patients may present with tremor (often of a "wing-beating" variety), dysarthria, rigidity, bradykinesia, dystonia and psychiatric disturbances. A pathognomonic feature of the neuropsychiatric form of the disease is the presence of Kayser-Fleischer rings, a brownish discoloration of the peripheral cornea seen on slit lamp examination of the eyes. Any young patient presenting with an unexplained tremor, parkinsonism or abnormal movements should receive a screening evaluation for Wilson's disease. This includes a serum ceruloplasmin level, measurement of urinary copper, and an ophthalmologic examination. Treatment includes lowering the amount of copper in the diet, as well as use of a copper chelator, usually D-penicillamine. Wilson's disease is one of the few potentially devastating genetic diseases for which there are effective medical therapies. A high index of suspicion is required to diagnose this treatable disorder.

HALLERVORDEN-SPATZ SYNDROME is a disease of the young, from infancy to young adulthood. Most cases are thought to be transmitted by autosomal recessive inheritance. Patients present with extrapyramidal symptoms including dystonia, rigidity, choreoathetosis and tremor, corticospinal tract signs, and dementia. The clinical course is progressive leading to death. Abnormal accumulation of iron has been found in the GP and SNr of affected individuals. This massive accumulation of iron often leads to prominent signal hypointensity in the GP and SNr on high field strength T2-weighted MRI. There is currently no effective treatment.

NEUROACANTHOCYTOSIS is characterized clinically by adult onset, progressive orofacial dyskinesia, chorea and dystonia of the limbs, and a predominantly motor polyneuropathy with amyotrophy[19]. Additional signs can include seizures, parkinsonism, areflexia, and variable psychiatric disturbances with or without dementia. Some patients experience a progressive akinetic-rigid syndrome that gradually replaces the hyperkinetic features[20]. It is usually transmitted by autosomal recessive inheritance although autosomal dominant, x-linked and sporadic cases have also been reported. Characteristic laboratory findings include increased levels of serum creatinine kinase and acanthocytes, erythrocytes with irregular spines projecting from the cell surface, presumably caused by a defect in membrane lipids. Pathology findings include atrophy of the caudate nuclei and putamena, and occasionally of the globi pallidi. Anterior horn cell loss may be present as well as chronic axonal neuropathy with demyelination[21]. Treatment is limited to symptomatic therapy with neuroleptics for chorea and anticonvulsants for seizures. Patients with bradykinesia or rigidity may respond to dopaminergic therapy.

HUNTINGTON'S DISEASE is a degenerative, autosomal-dominant disorder characterized by chorea, personality changes, and dementia[22]. Onset usually occurs in middle age, although some cases begin in childhood or adolescence[23]. Huntington's disease is caused by an increased number of trinucleotide (CAG) repeats in the gene on the short arm of chromosome 4[24]. The worldwide prevalence is 5-10 per 100,000. There is no therapy known to slow the progression of the disease and death commonly occurs 15-20 years after onset of symptoms.

Family members may notice that an affected patient has become short-tempered and depressed. He or she may be unable to sit still for any period of time, and may develop involuntary movements of the limbs, with decreased ocular saccades. Eventually, full choreiform movements develop, along with features of subcortical dementia. Atrophy of the caudate and putamen may be seen on imaging studies. Suicide is fairly common if depression emerges, and patients are usually confined to a nursing home in the later stages. Therapy is limited to symptomatic treatment using antidepressants for depression and neuroleptics when necessary to control chorea [25]. Neuroleptics can reduce chorea but often at the expense of side effects including apathy, sedation, akathisia, and parkinsonism. They should be reserved for those patients in whom chorea impairs function or self-care.

Five to ten percent of patients have juvenile Huntington's disease with onset before age twenty. Juvenile Huntington's disease is usually manifest by parkinsonian symptoms including bradykinesia, rigidity, and sometimes tremor. Dystonia and impaired eye movements may predominate and patients may have seizures. Ninety percent of juvenile Huntington's disease patients inherit the gene from an affected father, due to the large increase in the number of triplet repeats that can occur during spermatogenesis. Bradykinesia and rigidity may improve with levodopa therapy.

What are the "atypical parkinsonisms"?

The atypical parkinsonisms are a group of adult-onset progressive neurologic disorders that are characterized by bradykinesia and rigidity clinically and more widespread neuronal degeneration than Parkinson's disease histologically. The atypical parkinsonisms include progressive supranuclear palsy, corticobasal degeneration, and the multiple system atrophies. The multiple system atrophies are a group of closely related disorders that include degeneration in the extrapyramidal, pyramidal, autonomic and cerebellar systems.

How can I clinically recognize the atypical parkinsonisms?

In contrast to Parkinson's disease, the atypical parkinsonisms are generally symmetric, lack resting tremor, and respond little, if at all, to dopaminergic medications. There is usually early speech and balance impairment, and rigidity may be greater in the neck than the extremities. Some of the

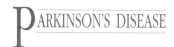

atypical parkinsonisms are associated with characteristic clinical signs that aid in their identification. The most important diagnostic distinction is between Parkinson's disease, which responds well to medical therapy, and the atypical parkinsonisms which do not.

What is progressive supranuclear palsy?

Progressive supranuclear palsy (PSP) is one of the atypical parkinsonisms or "parkinson plus" syndromes. It was originally described by Steele, Richardson, and Olszewski[26], and has a prevalence of approximately 7/100,000 individuals over age 55[27]. PSP has a later mean age of onset than Parkinson's disease, and most patients are in their sixties or seventies.

PSP is marked by bradykinesia and rigidity, postural instability, dysarthria, gait disturbances, and speech and swallowing difficulty[28]. Tremor is unusual. The characteristic clinical sign of PSP is a supranuclear gaze palsy. Downgaze is first affected followed by upgaze and later horizontal gaze. Slow saccade velocity may precede limitations of eye movements[28]. Some patients may complain of difficulty looking down, or note blurred vision but many have no visual complaints. Blink rate is markedly reduced and there may be "ocular stare" with the upper eyelids resting above the irises. Some patients exhibit neck extension rather than the stooped posture of Parkinson's disease. When turning, they may cross their feet rather than turning "en bloc" as do Parkinson's disease patients. Falling due to imbalance occurs relatively early. Blepharospasm and other focal dystonias are not unusual[29]. Dementia similar to that seen in patients with frontal lobe dysfunction is relatively common, particularly later in the disease[30]. On pathology examination, neuronal degeneration is present in the pallidum, subthalamic nucleus, and other areas. Lewy bodies are absent.

What are the multiple-system atrophies?

The multiple-system atrophies (MSAs) include striatonigral degeneration, Shy-Drager syndrome, and olivopontocerebellar atrophy[31,32]. Neuronal degeneration is much more widespread than in Parkinson's disease, and may include the striatum, substantia nigra, olives, pons, cerebellum, and spinal cord[32]. Lewy bodies are absent. Clinical symptoms of basal ganglia dysfunction, as well as cerebellar and autonomic dysfunction may be present. The early onset of frequent falling, coupled with cerebellar, pyramidal, or autonomic dysfunction usually suggests a diagnosis of MSA.

Resting tremor is unusual but may be seen in some cases. Speech is more severely affected in MSA than in Parkinson's disease, and patients often develop early and dramatic hypophonia. Abnormal eye movements consisting of slow saccades or impaired convergence may be present. Myoclonic jerks may also occur. Response to dopaminergic therapy is poor and treatment consists of symptomatic and supportive care.

What is Shy-Drager syndrome?

Shy-Drager syndrome is an atypical parkinsonism characterized by prominent autonomic dysfunction. Clinical features of autonomic dysfunction may include orthostatic hypotension (or syncope), impotence, urinary incontinence and sweating abnormalities. Vocal cord paralysis, speech disturbances, sleep apnea, and psychiatric changes may also occur.

G. Milton Shy and Glenn Drager originally described a group of patients with orthostatic hypotension, urinary incontinence, loss of sweating, ocular palsies, iris atrophy, rigidity, impotence, and wasting of distal musculature with EMG findings suggestive of anterior horn cell involvement [33]. The disorder most commonly affects patients in their 50s to 70s, and is more common in men. Impotence is a common early manifestation in men, while lightheadedness is often the first noticed feature in women. The disease is progressive, and ultimately leads to death.

On pathology, marked gliosis is seen in the intermediolateral column of the spinal cord with changes noted in sympathetic ganglia. Cell degeneration is also seen in the inferior olivary nucleus, dorsal vagus nucleus, and substantia nigra pars compacta. Abnormalities may be seen in the cerebellum, Edinger-Westphal nucleus, oculomotor nucleus, and caudate nucleus. Noradrenergic neurons of brain and sympathetic ganglia are affected, with marked loss of tyrosine hydroxylase activity in the locus ceruleus. Dopamine-β-hydroxylase activity has also found to be diminished in sympathetic ganglia [34].

Dopaminergic medications are usually not of benefit and may worsen symptoms of orthostasis [35]. Symptomatic therapy for orthostatic hypotension may be helpful.

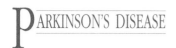

What is olivopontocerebellar atrophy?

Olivopontocerebellar atrophy (OPCA) is characterized by parkinsonism and cerebellar dysfunction [36]. The disease may occur by autosomal dominant inheritance or sporadically, and may affect individuals from infancy through the sixth decade. Patients may present with gait ataxia, extrapyramidal and pyramidal signs, and sphincter disturbances. Familial cases usually begin at a younger age, progress more slowly, and exhibit less autonomic failure than sporadic cases. Cerebellar abnormalities are usually the presenting feature of dominantly inherited forms of OPCA. Parkinsonian symptoms may be early or late manifestations [37]. Speech difficulties, swallowing impairment, dementia, and visual disturbances may also occur. Response to dopaminergic therapy is usually poor. Neuronal degeneration occurs in the pons, inferior olives, and cerebellar cortex as well as the substantia nigra, pyramidal tracts, and thalamus [38]. CT and MRI typically show cerebellar atrophy, with widened cerebellopontine cisterns [39].

What is striatonigral degeneration?

Striatonigral degeneration [40] is an adult-onset progressive, symmetric, bradykinetic-rigid disorder. It is characterized by early falling, speech and swallowing difficulties. Hyperreflexia and sleep apnea may be present. Resting tremor is much less common than in Parkinson's disease, and response to dopaminergic therapy is poor. Age at onset is comparable to that of Parkinson's disease, but progression of disability is much more rapid. On Pathology, neuronal loss is found in the striatum, with widespread changes also noted elsewhere [41,42]. Cell loss is also seen in the substantia nigra, but Lewy bodies are rare.

What is corticobasal ganglionic degeneration?

Corticobasal ganglionic degeneration is a progressive, adult-onset bradykinetic-rigid syndrome characterized by the presence of both parkinsonism and cortical dysfunction. In contrast to other atypical parkinsonisms, there is often marked asymmetry. Parkinsonian features include bradykinesia and asymmetric limb rigidity. Cortical features include apraxia and cortical sensory loss [43,44]. Patients may have involuntary mirror movements or levitation of an arm ("alien-limb" phenomenon). Associated features include postural instability, hyperreflexia, focal reflex myoclonus, and apraxia of eye movement. On Pathology the disease is characterized by asymmetric atrophy of the frontal and parietal lobes, and substantia nigra with neuronal achromasia [45]. There is no treatment known to be effective for this disorder.

What is diffuse Lewy body disease?

Diffuse Lewy body disease is a recently described atypical parkinsonism characterized by dementia, and autonomic abnormalities. It is marked pathologically by cortical and brainstem Lewy bodies [46, 47]. Symptoms may include fluctuations in cognitive state, depression, hallucinations, and paranoid delusions. Dementia usually occurs early in the disease, and parkinsonian features follow. Dysphasia and agnosia may also occur. On Pathology, Lewy bodies are found in the cortex, limbus, hypothalamus, and brainstem nuclei. The disease usually does not respond to dopamine replacement therapy.

PARKINSON'S DISEASE

CHAPTER 4

ETIOLOGY OF PARKINSON'S DISEASE

Although the exact cause of Parkinson's disease is unknown, research continues to provide clues as to possible etiologies. MPTP, a synthetic heroin byproduct which caused parkinsonism in users in the 1980s, renewed interest in the idea that Parkinson's disease may be caused by an environmental toxin. Despite an ongoing search, no toxin has yet been identified as a cause of Parkinson's disease in "idiopathic" cases. In one family a gene causing Parkinson's disease has been mapped to chromosome 4. Genetic factors seem to play a role in some cases, but in most individuals the genetic contribution appears small. Parkinson's disease may be multifactorial in etiology, with genetic predisposition causing susceptibility to one or more environmental toxins. At the molecular level, there is evidence that oxidative stress may cause dopamine neuron cell death. This chapter will examine these and other possible etiologies of Parkinson's disease.

Does aging cause Parkinson's disease?

Parkinson's disease most often occurs in individuals over 55 years of age. Because the disease is most prevalent in the elderly, it has been theorized that factors associated with aging might cause the disease. In fact, there are some features common to both Parkinson's disease and aging. Many elderly individuals exhibit some degree of bradykinesia although other signs of Parkinsonism are absent. Pathology studies have documented a loss of neurons in the substantia nigra pars compacta and putamen with advancing age [1], as well as a decrease in the cross-sectional size of the midbrain [2]. The rate of decline of dopaminergic neurons in elderly persons has been estimated to be as high as 10% per decade [3,4]. Levels of tyrosine hydroxylase, the rate limiting enzyme in the synthesis of dopamine, also decrease with advancing age [2].

Nonetheless, aging does not appear to be the cause of Parkinson's disease for the following reasons:

1. Most of the elderly do not have clinical evidence of Parkinson's disease.

2. The majority of Parkinson's disease cases are diagnosed in the presenile period (before ages 65 to 70), rather than in the senile period [5].

3. The prevalence of Parkinson's disease has remained stable over the past decade despite the increased number of elderly persons [5].

4. Bradykinesia in elderly patients without Parkinson's disease is not alleviated by levodopa [6].

5. The rate of dopaminergic cell loss in idiopathic Parkinson's disease is greater than that accounted for by normal aging and the regional loss of dopamine neurons in aging differs from that seen in Parkinson's disease. Loss of dopamine neurons in the substantia nigra pars compacta in normal aging is greatest in the medial ventral and dorsal tiers. In Parkinson's disease, neuronal loss in greatest in the lateral ventral tier, followed by the medial ventral and dorsal tiers [4].

6. Neuronal loss is greater in the putamen than in the caudate in idiopathic Parkinson's disease but not normal aging [7].

7. PET scans performed on healthy adults from ages 27 through 76 fail to show an aging effect on the uptake of fluorodopa into the caudate or putamen [8].

Therefore, although aging may contribute to a loss of dopaminergic neurons, it does not provide an explanation for the pattern or rate of dopamine neuron loss in idiopathic Parkinson's disease. This does not exclude the possibility that age-related changes may enhance susceptibility to etiologic factors or permit their expression.

Is Parkinson's disease an inherited disorder?

Most cases of Parkinson's disease appear to be sporadic. However, several large families have been identified in whom the disease is inherited as an autosomal dominant trait with incomplete penetrance.

Between 6% and 41% of Parkinson's disease patients are reported to have an affected relative [9]. This is two to ten times the percentage reported for normal individuals. Twin studies have compared concordance rates between monozygotic (MZ) and dizygotic (DZ) pairs. A genetic mechanism would cause twice the concordance rate for MZ compared to DZ twins. Early reports revealed low concordance rates with small differences between MZ and DZ pairs. Ward et al. reported a 4.7% concordance rate in 43 MZ twin pairs and a 5.3% concordance rate in 19 DZ twin pairs [10].

However, a recent larger study found concordance rates among pairs in whom the first affected member developed symptoms before age 60 of 39% for MZ pairs and 11% for DZ pairs. There was no difference between MZ and DZ pairs among older-onset pairs. This suggests a strong genetic determinant in younger onset Parkinson's disease patients.

Positron emission tomography (PET) and other new modalities may be useful in detecting preclinical cases, leading to a more accurate assessment of concordance. In one PET study, 5 of 11 (45%) MZ pairs and 2 of 7 (29%) DZ pairs were concordant [11].

Is there a Parkinson's disease gene?

In one large family with autosomal dominant Parkinson's disease a gene has been mapped to chromosome 4 [12]. This family originated in the town of Contursi in the Salerno province of southern Italy and some members emigrated to the United States, Germany, and other countries [13]. The kindred consists of 592 members with 60 affected individuals, the largest familial cluster ever discovered. Linkage analysis was performed using DNA samples from 9 family members with the disease and 19 without. Genetic markers at location 4q21-q23 demonstrated linkage with the disease phenotype. In the future, the exact location of the gene, now designated PARK1, will be identified and the gene will be characterized.

The percentage of Parkinson's disease patients outside this family who carry the gene will then be determined. It seems unlikely that the same mutation in the same gene is responsible for most cases as few families have as high a prevalence of Parkinson's disease as this one. Nonetheless, this family demonstrates that a single gene defect can cause Parkinson's disease.

Tremendous advances are likely to be made as research unravels the mechanism by which this gene causes disease.

What is the role of viruses in the etiology of Parkinson's disease?

Suspicion that viruses might play a role in the pathogenesis of Parkinson's disease was fueled by the occurrence of postencephalitic Parkinsonism, following the outbreak of encephalitis lethargica from 1917 - 1926. However, there is no clear evidence linking idiopathic Parkinson's disease to a viral infection. Virology studies performed on brains of Parkinson's disease patients using electron microscopy and immunofluorescent studies have failed to detect viral particles or antibodies[14]. Several studies have demonstrated an increase in herpes simplex antibody levels in patients with Parkinson's disease[15] but a causal relationship seems unlikely.

A negative association between a history of measles before college and the occurrence of Parkinson's disease has been reported[16]. The interpretation of this finding is unclear. It might indicate that measles protects against the development of Parkinson's disease, that individuals who were sheltered from childhood illnesses might have an increased risk of Parkinson's disease, or that measles in adulthood might be a risk factor for Parkinson's disease. There is also a suggestion that patients born between 1900 and 1930 have a higher incidence of Parkinson's disease if born during years marked by influenza pandemics[17]. Despite these observations, evidence linking a viral etiology to the pathogenesis of Parkinson's disease is scant.

What is the oxidation hypothesis?

The oxidation hypothesis suggests that chemical reactions involving electron transfers may cause or contribute to progression in Parkinson's disease. The intrinsic oxidation hypothesis postulates that dopamine's oxidative metabolism leads to the formation of harmful free radicals (figure 4-1). Oxidation reactions normally take place in the body and play important roles in the production of high energy compounds. A molecule is "oxidized" when it donates an electron, and "reduced" when it receives an electron. Oxidation reactions may lead to the formation of free radicals, highly reactive and unstable molecules that contain an unpaired electron. Oxygen is technically a free radical but it contains two unpaired electrons spinning in opposite directions and therefore reacts poorly with most molecules.

Dopamine's oxidative metabolism leads to the formation of hydrogen peroxide (figure 4-2). Hydrogen peroxide is normally rapidly cleared by protective mechanisms including glutathione. If protective mechanisms are overwhelmed, hydrogen peroxide can be reduced to form the highly reactive hydroxyl free radical which can react with membrane lipids in the brain, leading to lipid peroxidation and cell damage (figure 4-3). The brain may be particularly vulnerable to oxidative damage due to its large oxygen consumption, fertile material for lipid peroxidation, and limited ability to regenerate [18].

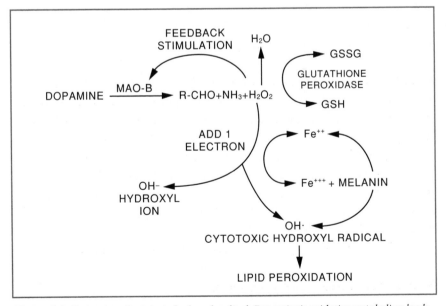

Figure 4-1. *Formation of cytotoxic hydroxyl radical. Dopamine's oxidative metabolism leads to the formation of hydrogen peroxide (H_2O_2). Hydrogen peroxide is normally cleared by glutathione. If protective mechanisms are overwhelmed, hydrogen peroxide can accept an electron to form hydroxyl ion (OH-) and cytotoxic hydroxyl radical (OH•). Melanin and iron may serve as electron donors and create site-specific oxidative stress.*

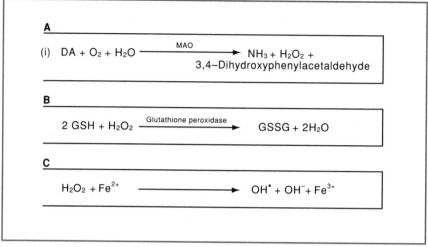

Figure 4-2. *A) Metabolism of dopamine by MAO. B) Clearance of H_2O_2 by reduced glutathione (GSH), thereby preventing the interaction of H_2O_2 with iron. C) The Fenton reaction. H_2O_2 that has not been cleared can accept an electron from Fe2+ to form the highly reactive hydroxyl radical (OH•).*

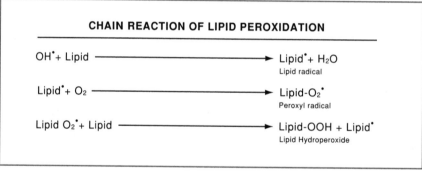

Figure 4-3. *The sequence of reactions in which the hydroxyl radical initiates lipid peroxidation.*

What is the evidence of oxidation reactions in Parkinson's disease?

The local environment of dopamine neurons may be particularly conducive to the formation of free radicals. One can predict that increased dopamine turnover, decreased protective mechanisms, and the presence of molecules that can donate electrons to facilitate oxidation reactions could promote free radical formation and damage due to lipid peroxidation. In Parkinson's disease there is increased dopamine turnover, decreased glutathione (a protective enzyme), increased iron (a transition metal that can readily transfer electrons), and evidence of increased lipid peroxidation.

Are protective enzymes decreased in Parkinson's disease?

Parkinson's disease patients have decreased levels of reduced glutathione in the substantia nigra, without an increase in oxidized glutathione [19]. These findings are thought to be specific to Parkinson's disease, and are not observed in conditions such as multiple system atrophy. It is unclear whether decreased glutathione levels are caused by abnormalities in its synthesis or metabolism and the exact localization of the deficiency is also unknown. Decreased levels of reduced glutathione may compromise protective mechanisms, allowing hydrogen peroxide to become available to form hydroxyl radicals.

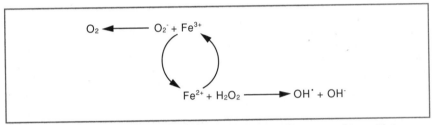

Figure 4-4. *Redox cycling of iron from its oxidized to its reduced state can drive oxidation reactions, thereby promoting the formation of cytotoxic free radicals.*

Is iron increased in Parkinson's disease?

Oxidation reactions are facilitated by transition metals including iron, copper, and manganese (figure 4-4). The brain contains a higher concentration of iron than any other metal, and it is probably essential for normal brain function. Iron accumulates in the normal brain until about age 20, after which time levels remain fairly constant. Iron is normally bound to the protein transferrin, which acts as a buffer to limit electron transfers. Parkinson's disease patients have increased iron levels in the substantia nigra pars compacta and decreased levels of transferrin, thus making iron more available for participation in oxidation reactions [20]. Melanin present in the substantia nigra has a high affinity for iron, and may serve as an electron source, thereby promoting the formation of free radicals [21]. The presence of neuromelanin may confer site specific vulnerability on substantia nigra neurons.

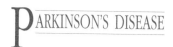

Is there evidence of increased lipid peroxidation?

Evidence of increased lipid peroxidation has been found in the substantia nigra of Parkinson's disease patients. There are higher levels of malondialdehyde, an intermediate in lipid peroxidation, and lipid hyperoxides [22]. Increased levels of thiobarbituric acid-reactive substances along with decreased levels of polyunsaturated fatty acids have also been observed.

What is the role of superoxide dismutase in Parkinson's disease?

Superoxide dismutase is a scavenger enzyme which may protect cells from free radical damage [23]. High levels of superoxide dismutase have been found in the substantia nigra on mitochondrial membranes of normal individuals [24]. Copper-zinc-dependent superoxide dismutase messenger RNA is higher in mesencephalic neurons containing neruomelanin compared to other neurons, suggesting that melanized neurons require a defense against free radicals [25]. Increased superoxide dismutase levels are found in Parkinson's disease patients irrespective of gender, age, or treatment [26]. This may reflect an effort to defend against increased free radical production.

What is MPTP?

MPTP, or 1-methyl-4-phenyl-1,2,3,6-tetrahydropyridine, causes a clinical syndrome closely mimicking idiopathic Parkinson's disease. This was first observed in a chemist who was synthesizing illicit substances in his lab. He developed Parkinsonism after intravenous injection of a mixture of 1-methyl-4-phenyl-4-hydroxypiperidine or MPPP, a potent meperidine analogue, and MPTP [27]. Autopsy revealed dopaminergic neuronal degeneration specifically within the substantia nigra. Several other individuals who self-injected MPTP were later identified and examined [28]. Shortly after intravenous injection, these patients developed visual hallucinations, stiffness, limb jerking, and immobility. This stage was also marked by a sense of euphoria and burning at the injection site. Bradykinesia progressed for up to three weeks after injection. The ensuing chronic stage was marked by all of the motor features of Parkinson's disease, as well as some infrequent findings including eyelid apraxia, freezing, and dystonia. Levodopa administration brought about marked improvement in Parkinsonian signs and symptoms, and side effects of chronic dopamine replacement therapy, including dyskinesia, occurred more rapidly than in idiopathic Parkinson's disease [28]. Autopsies revealed selective destruction of the dopaminergic neurons of the pars compacta of the substantia nigra. MPTP has since been utilized to create an excellent animal model of Parkinson's disease for research.

MPTP is actually a protoxin which is oxidized to the true toxin MPP+ by the enzyme monoamine oxidase type B (figure 4-5). MPP+ accumulates in mitochondria, and interferes with the function of Complex I of the respiratory chain. The extrinsic oxidation hypothesis suggests that an environmental protoxin is oxidized to a toxin that causes Parkinson's disease. Searches for such an environmental toxin have not identified a chemical that is likely to cause Parkinson's disease in idiopathic cases. Still, the identification of a chemical causing a syndrome so similar to Parkinson's disease is a landmark discovery which continues to provide new insights into possible etiologic mechanisms.

CH₃
|
N

Selegiline

MAO-B

CH₃
|
⁺N

MPTP
1-methyl-4-phenyl-1,2,3,6-
tetrahydropyridine

MPP+
1-methyl-4-
phenylpyridinium ion

Figure 4-5. *Oxidation of MPTP to MPP+ is inhibited by selegiline, a selective inhibitor of MAO-B.*

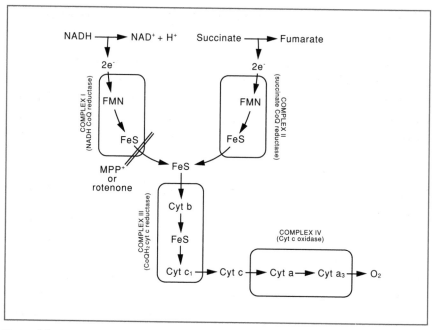

Figure 4-6. *MPP+ inhibits complex I of the respiratory chain.*

What is the role of mitochondria in the pathogenesis of Parkinson's disease?

The toxic metabolite of MPTP, MPP+ inhibits complex I of the electron transport chain, causing a parkinsonian syndrome in affected individuals and laboratory animals [29] (figure 4-6). This raises the question as to whether complex I is abnormal in idiopathic Parkinson's disease. Several laboratories have reported deficiencies of mitochondrial electron transport chain complex I in the substantia nigra of Parkinson's disease patients [30]. A blinded study examining platelet mitochondrial activity in early untreated Parkinson's disease patients and age-and sex-matched controls found lower complex I activity in platelet mitochondria in the former group [31]. This suggests that chemical defects in Parkinson's disease may be widely expressed in the body. Although complex I activity is diminished, no correlation with duration of disease has been found. In Parkinson-plus patients complex I activity is normal [32].

What is the role of smoking in the etiology of Parkinson's disease?

Cigarette smokers have been reported to have a lower risk of developing Parkinson's disease than non-smokers[33]. The most plausible explanation for this observation is that smoking causes an induction of protective enzymes, but this is unproven. No benefit is known to accrue to Parkinson's disease patients who smoke and they should be advised to quit for general health reasons just like any other patient.

What is the role of neurotrophic factors in Parkinson's disease?

It has been suggested that neurodegenerative disorders may result from a lack of disorder-specific neurotrophic factors. Thus far, however, no deficiency of a neurotrophic factor has been causally linked to a disease state. On the other hand, neurotrophic factors are capable of increasing neuronal survival, protecting neurons against injury, and promoting the sprouting of dopaminergic axons[34]. This has raised the possibility of using trophic factors to prevent or slow further dopamine neuron degeneration in Parkinson's disease.

Several neurotrophic growth factors have recently been cloned. One of these is glial cell line-derived neurotrophic factor or GDNF, which was found to prolong the survival of dopaminergic neurons in embryonic midbrain cultures[35]. BDNF, or brain-derived neurotrophic factor[36] has also been shown to increase the survival of dopaminergic neurons. Neurotrophin-4/5 has recently been shown to prevent death of rat dopaminergic neurons in culture, and can protect dopaminergic neurons of embryos from the toxic effects of MPP+ [37].

One of the difficulties of developing trophic factors as a treatment for Parkinson's disease is that they do not readily cross the blood-brain barrier. Various delivery systems are now under investigation and trophic factors may hold much promise for the future.

PARKINSON'S DISEASE

CHAPTER 5

MEDICATIONS FOR THE TREATMENT OF PARKINSON'S DISEASE

When did the modern era of Parkinson's disease treatment begin?

The discovery that Parkinson's disease is associated with a striatal dopamine deficiency created new possibilities for therapeutic approaches beginning in the late 1960s. Until then, anticholinergic medications were the principal treatment and results were disappointing. Patients were subsequently found to experience dramatic benefit when placed on the dopamine precursor, levodopa [1]. Today, levodopa therapy remains the gold standard of symptomatic treatment for Parkinson's disease. However, long-term therapy with levodopa is less than satisfactory as disability continues to progress and most patients develop levodopa-associated motor fluctuations and dyskinesia within a few years of treatment. Many patients ultimately develop disability due to difficulty with balance and cognition. For this reason, much research in Parkinson's disease today focuses on how to forestall disability and maintain or improve function over the long-term.

What are the basic categories of therapies used to treat Parkinson's disease?

Treatments are potentially divided into those that are: a) symptomatic, b) neuroprotective, and c) restorative.

Symptomatic therapies are those that improve signs and symptoms without affecting the underlying disease state. Degeneration of the substantia nigra in Parkinson's disease causes a striatal dopamine deficiency. Administration of levodopa increases dopamine concentration in the striatum, especially when its peripheral metabolism is inhibited by a peripheral decarboxylase inhibitor (PDI). Levodopa/PDI therapy is currently the gold standard of symptomatic therapy for Parkinson's disease. Catechol-O-methyltransferase (COMT) inhibitors further inhibit levodopa's peripheral metabolism, thereby enhancing central bioavailability. Selegiline increases dopamine activity in the brain by inhibiting its metabolism. Dopamine agonists provide symptomatic benefit by directly stimulating post-synaptic striatal dopamine receptors. Other medications used in the treatment of Parkinson's disease include amantadine, which augments dopamine release and anticholinergics such as trihexyphenidyl and benztropine, which block striatal cholinergic function. Each of these medications is discussed in greater detail below.

Neuroprotective therapies are those that slow neuronal degeneration, thereby delaying disease progression. Recent interest has focused on selegiline, a monoamine oxidase-B inhibitor. Selegiline inhibits the oxidative metabolism of levodopa and may reduce oxidative stress and free radical formation. New neurotrophic factors are now being evaluated for their ability to slow disease progression.

Restorative therapies are those that aim to replace lost neurons. One approach to replacing lost neurons is the transplantation of embryonic tissue. Transplanted embryonic tissue may survive, restore neuronal connections, increase dopamine concentration and improve function. Genetically engineered cells, animal dopaminergic cells, and cells from other parts of the human body are being developed for transplantation and may also have restorative effects.

What is levodopa?

Levodopa is the chemical precursor of dopamine. The dopamine depletor reserpine was found to produce parkinsonian symptoms in rats in the late 1950s[2]. In addition, post-mortem examinations of Parkinson's disease patients revealed decreased dopamine concentration in the striatum, correlating with the loss of nigro-striatal neurons in the substantia nigra[3]. As dopamine does not cross the blood-brain barrier, its precursor, levodopa, was tested as dopamine replacement therapy. Parkinson's disease patients were soon treated with levodopa with convincing results[4]. The main difficulty with early levodopa preparations was the high incidence of nausea and vomiting. Peripheral decarboxylase inhibitors were found to improve the clinical utility of levodopa by reducing its peripheral breakdown[5]. Decreased peripheral dopamine production reduced the incidence of nausea and vomiting and allowed more levodopa to cross the blood-brain barrier. The decarboxylase inhibitors carbidopa and benserazide are most commonly combined with levodopa for this purpose.

What are the pharmacokinetics of levodopa?

Levodopa, or l-dihydroxyphenylalanine, is a large neutral amino acid. After oral ingestion, it is absorbed in the proximal small intestine by a saturable, carrier-mediated transport system. Absorption can be delayed by meals[6] and increased gastric acidity[7]. Absorbed levodopa is not bound to plasma protein and its half-life is approximately one hour[8]. To exert an anti-parkinsonian effect, levodopa must cross the blood-brain barrier by way of the large neutral amino acid carrier transport system.

What is levodopa/carbidopa?

Levodopa/carbidopa is a combination of carbidopa, a peripheral decarboxylase inhibitor, and levodopa. Carbidopa lessens the extracerebral decarboxylation of levodopa, thereby decreasing the incidence of nausea and increasing the central availability of levodopa. The addition of carbidopa reduces the amount of levodopa needed by about 75%[9]. Approximately 75 to 100 mg of carbidopa are required to saturate peripheral decarboxylase[5]. Nonetheless, some patients require carbidopa in doses up to 200 mg per day to reduce or eliminate nausea. The half-life of levodopa when administered with carbidopa is approximately two and a half hours[9]. Standard levodopa/carbidopa is usually administered one half hour or more before, or one hour or more after meals to achieve the most consistent absorption. Although levodopa competes with other large, neutral amino acids for transport across the blood-brain barrier, only patients with meaningful motor fluctuations on levodopa/PDI need consider a low/balanced protein or protein redistributed diet.

How do I initiate levodopa therapy?

A commonly used initial target dose is carbidopa/levodopa 25/100 TID, starting with half of a 25/100 tablet each day for the first week and increasing by a half tablet per day each week until the target dose is reached. The final dose must be tailored to the individual patient.

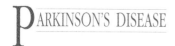

What are the side effects of levodopa/PDI?

The most common side effect of levodopa/PDI is nausea. This is due to stimulation of the vomiting center in the medulla by dopamine formed peripherally. If a patient has difficulty initiating levodopa/PDI due to nausea, he may take it with a carbohydrate snack or immediately following a meal. Additional carbidopa may be helpful if nausea persists and is available directly from the manufacturer. These steps will allow the vast majority of patients to tolerate levodopa/PDI without much difficulty. Where available, the use of a peripherally acting neuroleptic, such as domperidone is very helpful to alleviate refractory nausea due to levodopa.

Other potential side effects of levodopa/PDI include orthostatic hypotension, confusion, hallucinations, delusions, and hypersexuality. Orthostatic hypotension can usually be countered with fludrocortisone or midodrine [10]. Cognitive side effects typically occur later in the disease in patients who have developed underlying dementia. Confusion may improve with a decrease in levodopa dose. Hallucinations and delusions can be treated with clozapine, an atypical neuroleptic with minimal parkinsonian side effects (see below).

What is levodopa/carbidopa CR?

Levodopa/carbidopa CR is a controlled-release preparation. It is more slowly absorbed and provides more sustained serum levels than standard levodopa/carbidopa [11]. It is best absorbed when taken with food and levodopa bioavailability is about 80% that of standard levodopa/carbidopa [12]. One potential drawback is that it takes about a half an hour longer to begin to exert its effect. The initial target dose is carbidopa/levodopa CR 25/100 TID or 50/200 BID, usually starting with 100 mg levodopa per day and slowly increasing. To convert a patient from standard levodopa/carbidopa to levodopa/carbidopa CR, the daily dosage is increased by approximately 20% while the number of daily doses is decreased by 30-50% [13,14].

When I begin levodopa should I use standard levodopa/carbidopa or levodopa/carbidopa CR?

Standard and CR levodopa/carbidopa are equally effective in improving motor symptoms when levodopa is first required. CR is often more convenient because fewer daily doses are required. In addition, there is interest as to whether more stable dopamine receptor stimulation as afforded by levodopa/carbidopa CR can forestall the development of long-term complications including motor fluctuations and dyskinesia. However, a five year study comparing standard and CR levodopa/carbidopa found no difference in the incidence of fluctuations and dyskinesia [15]. Nonetheless, functional scores (Activities of Daily Living) were significantly more improved in patients taking CR levodopa/carbidopa.

What are the side effects of levodopa/carbidopa CR?

Side effects of levodopa/carbidopa CR are similar to those of standard levodopa/carbidopa, but they may take a longer time to dissipate. Thus, patients with dyskinesia may experience more dyskinesia when switched to levodopa/carbidopa CR. In our experience, some patients with nausea may benefit from a switch from standard to CR or vice versa and one cannot predict which will cause less nausea in a given patient. Patients with moderate disease often need a small amount of standard levodopa/carbidopa as part of the first morning dose to act as a "booster" and bring on symptomatic benefit more quickly. This is often accomplished by adding one carbidopa/levodopa 25/100 tablet to the first CR dose of the day.

What is levodopa/benserazide HBS?

Levodopa/benserazide hydrodynamically balanced system (HBS) is a controlled-release levodopa preparation containing hydrocolloids, fats, and the decarboxylase inhibitor benserazide. Levodopa/benserazide HBS "floats" on stomach contents for five to twelve hours allowing levodopa to be slowly absorbed. Compared to standard levodopa/benserazide, levodopa bioavailability is about 60%, so a switch usually necessitates a dosage increase [16]. As with other controlled-release preparations, it is often supplemented with a small dose of the standard formulation to provide an early morning "kick".

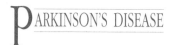

What symptoms of Parkinson's disease are best alleviated by levodopa therapy?

Levodopa therapy is the cornerstone of symptomatic treatment. It is most effective in relieving bradykinesia and rigidity, while its effect on tremor is highly variable [17]. Balance difficulty is not effectively alleviated by levodopa.

When assessing the benefit of levodopa, one should evaluate motor function, bradykinesia and rigidity. Symptomatic improvement may or may not occur if a patient only has tremor. In addition, improvement may be difficult to detect if symptoms are minimal. Improvement with levodopa therapy is usually apparent with more advanced disease as motor dysfunction, bradykinesia, and rigidity become more obvious.

What are dopamine agonists?

Dopamine agonists directly stimulate post-synaptic dopamine receptors [18]. They provide symptomatic benefit as adjuncts to levodopa, and as monotherapy in early disease. There is interest as to whether their early and sustained use can forestall long-term levodopa-associated complications. Monotherapy with dopamine agonists is generally as effective as levodopa/PDI when a patient first requires symptomatic therapy [19,20]. After one to three years of disease progression, monotherapy with a dopamine agonist often becomes inadequate and levodopa therapy must be added. In moderate and advanced disease, patients with motor fluctuations on levodopa may benefit from the addition of a dopamine agonist to smooth motor fluctuations and improve symptom control.

What are the side effects of dopamine agonists?

Dopamine agonists can cause nausea, vomiting, and orthostatic hypotension by stimulating peripheral dopamine receptors. They may also cause central dopaminergic side effects such as nightmares, hallucinations, or psychiatric symptoms. Cognitive side effects are dose related but nausea and orthostatic hypotension can occur even with small initial doses. Other possible side effects include leg edema and constipation [21].

Should dopamine agonists be given with or without food?

Meals have little effect on the extent of absorption of dopamine agonists and they can be taken with or without food. Patients with nausea should take their medication after a meal. For patients on combination therapy with levodopa, the dopamine agonist is usually scheduled to be taken when levodopa is administered as a matter of convenience.

What is bromocriptine?

Bromocriptine is an ergot alkaloid dopamine receptor agonist (figure 5-1). It is a strong D2 receptor agonist and a weak D1 receptor antagonist (5-2). It stimulates both pre- and post-synaptic receptors, and its half-life is approximately seven hours [9]. It can be initiated at a dose of one half of a 2.5 mg tablet per day, and increased slowly to a daily dose in the range of 10-40 mg per day [21]. Potential side effects include nausea, vomiting, orthostatic hypotension, confusion, hallucinations, anorexia, and erythromelalgia, a painful, reddish discoloration of the skin. Retroperitoneal fibrosis has been reported in a few patients who received long-term therapy at daily dosages of 30-140 mg.

| | Receptor Binding | | | | | |
	D_2	D_3	D_1	$5HT_{1/2}$	α_1	α_2
Bromocriptine[1]	++	+	+	++	++	++
Pergolide[2]	++	++	++	++	+	++
Ropinirole	++	+++	-	-	-	-
Pramipexole	++	+++	-	-	-	-

[1] Bromocriptine is a D_1 Antagonist   [2] Pergolide is a D_1 Agonist

Figure 5-2. *Receptor binding of bromocriptine, pergolide, ropinirole and pramipexole.*

What is pergolide?

Pergolide is a semisynthetic, clavine ergot derivative dopamine agonist (figure 5-1). In contrast to bromocriptine, it is a strong D2 receptor agonist and a weak D1 receptor agonist (figure 5-2). Peak plasma levels are achieved in one to two hours, and its half-life is approximately 20-27 hours [9]. The starting dose is half of a 0.05 mg tablet per day, with an initial target dose of 0.25 mg TID achieved over one month. Daily doses of up to 3.0 mg per day in divided doses are usually well tolerated. Potential side effects include nausea, vomiting, orthostatic hypotension, cognitive dysfunction, increased liver enzymes, erythromelalgia, and peripheral edema [23].

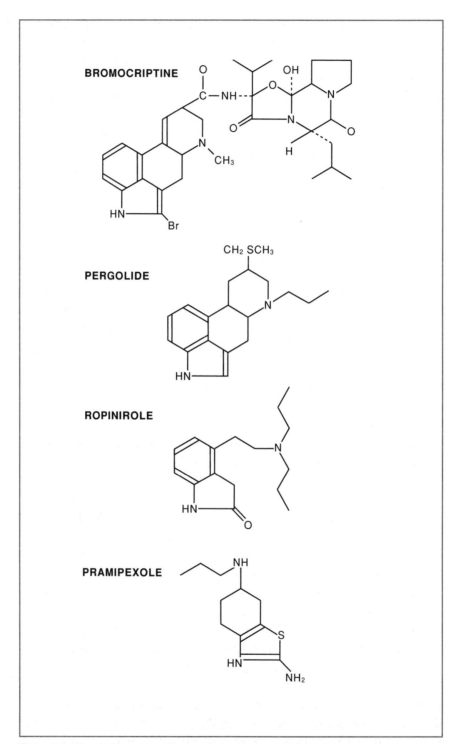

Figure 5-1. *Chemical structures of bromocriptine and pergolide, ropinirole and pramipexole.*

Pergolide was compared to placebo as an adjunct to levodopa in patients with motor fluctuations[24]. Pergolide permitted a mean levodopa dose reduction of 24.7% compared with 4.9% in the placebo group (p < .001). Motor function improved by 35% in pergolide-treated patients compared with 17% in placebo-treated patients (p < .001) and "off" time decreased by 32% compared with 4% (p < .001). Although new onset or worsening of dyskinesia was observed in 62% of the pergolide group compared to 25% of the placebo group during the study, dyskinesia was generally controlled by a reduction of levodopa dose such that there was no difference in dyskinesia disability by the end of the study.

What is ropinirole?

Ropinirole is a potent, highly selective D2 agonist with little affinity for D1, 5HT, muscarinic, or adrenergic receptors (figure 5-2). It is a non-ergoline dopamine agonist and has a half-life of approximately six hours (figure 5-1). Maximal plasma concentration is reached approximately 1.5 hours after administration in fasted patients and approximately 4 hours when taken with meals[25]. The starting dose is 0.25 mg TID, with an initial target dose of 1 mg TID achieved over one month. Many patients respond to a dose of 1-3 mg TID with further titration undertaken as clinically necessary. Doses of up to 8 mg TID have been studied. Side effects are similar to other dopamine agonists and include nausea, somnolence, insomnia, dizziness, dyspepsia, and headache[21]. Ergot-related pleural and retroperitoneal fibrosis have not been reported.

Ropinirole is effective both as early monotherapy and as an adjunct to treatment with levodopa. A number of well-controlled, double-blind, prospective clinical trials have confirmed the safety and efficacy of ropinirole in the treatment of Parkinson's disease. One study compared ropinirole to placebo as add-on therapy in patients not optimally controlled on levodopa. At six months, 27.7% of ropinirole-treated patients had at least a 20% reduction in levodopa dose *and* at least a 20% reduction in "off" time compared with 11% in the placebo group (odds ratio = 4.4; 95% confidence interval, 1.53 to 12.66)[26]. Mean reduction of levodopa dose in the ropinirole group was 19.4%.

In a study of ropinirole as monotherapy in early stage patients, motor function was improved by 24% at six months in ropinirole-treated patients compared with a 3% worsening in placebo treated patients (p < .001)[27]. Significantly fewer ropinirole-treated patients required "rescue" with

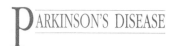

levodopa compared with placebo-treated patients (11% vs. 29%, p < 0.001). In a six month study comparing ropinirole with levodopa in early stage patients, a similar percentage of patients in each group experienced greater than 30% improvement (48% vs. 58%), although levodopa-treated patients experienced significantly greater improvement overall (32% vs. 44%) [20].

Ropinirole has been demonstrated to be more effective than bromocriptine as monotherapy in patients who are not taking selegiline. In a six-month study comparing ropinirole with bromocriptine as early monotherapy, ropinirole brought about significantly greater improvement (34%) than bromocriptine (20%) [28]. Benefit was similar in selegiline-treated patients as selegiline appeared to enhance the efficacy of bromocriptine to the level of ropinirole.

What is pramipexole?

Pramipexole is a non-ergot D2/D3 agonist (figure 5-2). It is a synthetic amino-benzathiazol derivative that binds to D3 receptors with 7-fold greater affinity than to D2 or D4 receptors and has little affinity for D1, 5HT, muscarinic, or adrenergic receptors [29]. Pramipexole is introduced at a dose of 0.25 mg/day and escalated to an initial target of 1.5 mg/day over approximately one month. The usual maximum dose is 3 to 4.5 mg/day. Side effects are similar to other dopamine agonists and include somnolence, nausea, constipation, insomnia, and hallucinations [30,31]. Somnolence may be more common than with other dopaminergic medications and may necessitate dose reduction or discontinuation. Ergot-related pleural and retroperitoneal fibrosis have not been reported.

Pramipexole is effective both as early monotherapy and as an adjunct to treatment with levodopa. In a six month trial comparing pramipexole to placebo as add-on therapy in patients with motor fluctuations on levodopa, "off" time was reduced by 17% in pramipexole-treated patients compared with 8% in placebo-treated patients (p < .01) [31]. Levodopa was reduced by 25% in the pramipexole group compared with 6% in the placebo group (p < .01). Pramipexole significantly improved motor function in both the "on" and "off" states. In a comparison of pramipexole to placebo as monotherapy in early disease, pramipexole significantly improved motor function (p < .0001) [30].

What is cabergoline?

Cabergoline is a long-acting ergot derivative agonist [32] with a high affinity for D2 receptors [33]. Its biological half-life is approximately sixty-five hours [34] and it is usually administered as a once a day dose. Cabergoline can be introduced at a dose of 0.05 mg and titrated to a usual maximum of 5 mg once daily. Side effects are similar to other agonists and include dizziness, hypersomnolence, headache, nausea, and orthostatic hypotension [35].

In a six month study comparing cabergoline to placebo as adjunctive therapy to levodopa for patients with motor fluctuations, cabergoline allowed an 18% reduction in levodopa dose compared with 3% in placebo-treated patients (p < .001) [36]. Motor function improved 16% in the cabergoline group compared with 6% in the control group (p = .031). "On" time was significantly increased (p = .02) and associated with a corresponding decrease in "off" time and "on time with dyskinesia".

Are there other dopamine agonists?

Lisuride is a hydrophilic semisynthetic ergot alkaloid dopamine agonist. It stimulates D2 and 5-HT (serotonin) receptors [37]. When given orally its half-life is 1.5 to 2 hours. It is water-soluble and can also be administered subcutaneously or by continuous intravenous infusion to help ameliorate severe motor fluctuations [38, 39].

Apomorphine is a D2 and D1 receptor agonist. It is highly lipophilic and usually administered subcutaneously. Onset of action is within five to fifteen minutes and its effect lasts 90 to 120 minutes [40]. Because of its rapid onset of action, it can be used as a rescue agent for refractory off periods. Its use is limited by prominent side effects including nausea, vomiting, and azotemia. Anti-emetics such as domperidone may be helpful to reduce associated nausea and vomiting [41,42].

What are the advantages of using dopamine agonists?

There are two main concerns regarding possible harm from chronic levodopa therapy: 1) dopamine's oxidative metabolism may lead to free radical formation and cause or accelerate neuronal degeneration, and 2) rapidly fluctuating levels of levodopa-derived dopamine may sensitize dopamine receptors and lead to dyskinesia. Unlike levodopa, dopamine agonists directly stimulate post-synaptic dopamine receptors. They do not undergo oxidative metabolism and there is no concern that they might accelerate the disease process. In fact, animals fed a diet including pergolide were found to experience less age-related loss of dopamine neurons [43]. Bromocriptine, pergolide, ropinirole, pramipexole, and cabergoline all have significantly longer half-lives than levodopa and do not expose receptors to rapidly fluctuating levels of stimulation. Animal studies have demonstrated that dopamine agonists are associated with a lower incidence of dyskinesia than levodopa [44]. Several investigators have examined the possibility that dopamine agonists, alone or in combination with levodopa, could delay motor fluctuations and dyskinesia. A series of retrospective studies found fewer motor complications in patients treated with agonists rather than levodopa [45]. In addition, several prospective studies have found that initial treatment with a dopamine agonist followed by the addition of levodopa when necessary is associated with a lower prevalence of dyskinesia [46,47].

The main limitation of dopamine agonist monotherapy is that symptoms are adequately controlled for a period of only one to three years. Rinne found that after three years of bromocriptine monotherapy only 28%, and after 5 years only 7%, of patients were still adequately maintained on monotherapy alone [48]. After a few years, most patients require levodopa to sustain good benefit.

In moderate and advanced disease, dopamine agonists provide benefit for patients with motor fluctuations on levodopa therapy. When an agonist is added, off time is reduced, motor function is improved and levodopa doses may be reduced. Only rarely can a patient with fluctuations and dyskinesia be adequately managed with dopamine agonists alone.

How do I switch from one agonist to another?

One can switch directly from one agonist to another by substituting potency equivalent doses. Alternatively, a patient can be tapered off one agonist before introducing another at a low dose and escalating upward. The mg potency ratio of bromocriptine to pergolide is approximately 10:1. Therefore a patient on 20 mg of bromocriptine per day can usually be switched directly to 2 mg of pergolide per day. There is limited information currently available concerning the relative mg potency ratios of the new dopamine agonists. Pramipexole and cabergoline may be dosed similarly to pergolide. The mg potency ratio of ropinirole to pergolide may be approximately 6:1.

Figure 5-3. *Chemical structures of selegiline, a selective MAO-B inhibitor; pargyline, a non-selective MAO inhibitor; and clorgyline, a selective MAO-A inhibitor.*

Can I abruptly stop dopaminergic medications?

The dopaminergic medications (levodopa preparations and the dopamine agonists) should generally not be abruptly discontinued. Although many patients will tolerate abrupt withdrawal without difficulty, there is the possibility that a rare patient may experience neuroleptic malignant syndrome, a potentially fatal condition.

What is selegiline?

Selegiline is a relatively selective, irreversible monoamine oxidase type B (MAO-B) inhibitor (figure 5-3). In the brain, MAO-B is partly responsible for the catabolism of dopamine. Selegiline boosts the symptomatic effect of levodopa by slowing the breakdown of levodopa-derived dopamine. In the research literature selegiline was known as deprenyl or l-deprenyl. The standard dose is 5 mg PO BID with breakfast and lunch.

How was selegiline created?

Selegiline was initially intended to be a "psychic energizer", created by combining an amphetamine moiety with an antidepressant-like compound[49]. The development of MAO inhibitors began in the 1950s, when iproniazid, an anti-tuberculosis agent, was found to improve depression. Early antidepressants were difficult to use as MAO-A inhibitors were associated with the risk of hypertensive crisis. Normally, MAO-A in the gut metabolizes ingested amines such as tyramine and prevents their absorption.

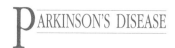

When MAO-A in the gut is inhibited, ingested amines can be absorbed and may cause sympathomimetic crises, sometimes called the "cheese effect". Manifestations of sympathomimetic crisis include hypertension, vomiting, increased heart rate, and headache. When gut MAO-A is inhibited, levodopa can cause sympathomimetic crisis as readily as tyramine. For this reason, levodopa preparations should not be given concurrently with MAO-A inhibitors. As a relatively selective MAO-B inhibitor, selegiline can be safely administered with levodopa. Selegiline is highly selective for inhibition of MAO-B in doses up to 10 mg per day [49]. It is unsafe to use higher selegiline doses with levodopa and for this reason almost all studies of selegiline in Parkinson's disease have employed a 10 mg per day dosage.

How long does selegiline's effect last?

When ingested orally, selegiline is absorbed and crosses the blood-brain barrier without difficulty. Its plasma half-life is almost 40 hours [50] and its functional half-life is longer. As a "suicide" inhibitor, selegiline forms a covalent bond with MAO and restoration of MAO function is dependent on the generation of new enzyme. A selegiline effect probably persists for three to four months after its discontinuation.

What are the side effects of selegiline?

Selegiline is generally very well tolerated. Because it is metabolized to amphetamine derivatives, it is typically administered in the morning and at midday rather than in the evening to minimize the potential for insomnia. Some patients experience gastrointestinal side effects. Unusual side effects include increased liver enzymes and aggravation of peptic ulcer disease [51]. When administered concurrently with levodopa, the most common side effect is an exacerbation of dopaminergic adverse effects. If a patient has peak-dose dyskinesias or hallucinations on levodopa, these may worsen with the addition of selegiline [52]. The physician should then lower the levodopa dose to alleviate these symptoms. For patients who have side effects on levodopa/PDI alone, it may be helpful to introduce selegiline at a low dose (one half tablet). This will allow an opportunity to reduce the levodopa dose in response to a worsening of side effects as the selegiline dose is escalated. A reduction of levodopa/PDI of approximately 20% is often required.

What medications should be avoided in patients who are taking selegiline?

A constellation of symptoms known as the serotonin syndrome may occur with the use of serotomimetic agents, taken alone or in combination with MAO inhibitors including selegiline. These agents include serotonin reuptake inhibitors, tricyclic and tetracyclic antidepressants, meperidine and other opiates, dextromethorphan, and tryptophan. The syndrome is characterized by various combinations of confusion, agitation, restlessness, rigidity, hyperreflexia, shivering, autonomic instability, myoclonus, coma, low grade fever, nausea, diarrhea, diaphoresis, flushing, and rarely rhabdomyolysis and death [53]. Patients taking selegiline should therefore avoid meperidine and other opiates. The actual incidence of serious events when selegiline is used in combination with antidepressants is unclear. As many patients with Parkinson's disease suffer with depression, this issue raises difficult management questions. One chart review study did not identify any major side effects from combination therapy and serious interactions appear rare [54]. Nonetheless, it seems prudent to provide informed consent or discontinue selegiline prior to introducing these antidepressants.

When should I use selegiline?

Selegiline is beneficial as an adjunct to levodopa for patients who are experiencing a deterioration in the quality of their response. For patients with motor fluctuations, selegiline reduces "off" time and extends the short duration response of levodopa. In addition, there is interest in whether selegiline can slow progression of Parkinson's disease [55].

Why is there interest in whether selegiline can slow disease progression?

The concept that selegiline might slow disease progression initially came from three observations. The ability of the neurotoxin MPTP to cause dopamine cell death and induce parkinsonian symptoms in animals and man is dependent on its oxidation to MPP+ by MAO-B. When selegiline is administered prior to MPTP, MPTP is not converted to MPP+ and parkinsonian symptoms are not elicited [56]. If there is an environmental neurotoxin similar to MPTP that causes Parkinson's disease in man, then selegiline might prevent its oxidation and protect against dopamine cell damage. Similarly, if free radical formation from the oxidative metabolism

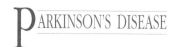

of dopamine by MAO-B contributes to disease progression, inhibition of MAO-B by selegiline may reduce free radical formation and slow dopamine cell degeneration. Finally, an early retrospective study found that patients on selegiline lived longer than those not on selegiline [57].

What is the DATATOP study?

The Parkinson Study Group examined the ability of selegiline and tocopherol (vitamin E), alone or together, to slow the progression of Parkinson's disease. This study was called "Deprenyl and Tocopherol Antioxidative Therapy of Parkinsonism", or DATATOP. Eight hundred patients with early Parkinson's disease not yet requiring levodopa therapy were enrolled in the study. Subjects were randomized to one of four groups in a 2 by 2 factorial design: 1) selegiline (10 mg/day) and tocopherol placebo, 2) tocopherol (2000 IU/day) and selegiline placebo, 3) selegiline and tocopherol, or 4) selegiline placebo and tocopherol placebo. The primary endpoint was the time required for the patient to develop sufficient disability to warrant the use of levodopa therapy. Results demonstrated that patients assigned to receive selegiline (alone or with tocopherol) experienced a significant delay in the need for levodopa therapy (hazard ratio = 0.50, p<0.001) (figure 5-4) [55]. Patients on selegiline placebo required levodopa at a projected median of 15 months from enrollment compared to 24 months for patients on selegiline. Tocopherol had no effect on the endpoint. This study conclusively demonstrates that the use of selegiline in early Parkinson's disease delays the need for levodopa therapy and is consistent with the hypothesis that selegiline may slow disease progression. However, the study also found that selegiline alone provided a small symptomatic benefit. One cannot the exclude the possibility that the delay in need for levodopa was due entirely or in part to this small symptomatic effect.

Are there studies that suggest selegiline may slow progression later in the disease?

One study evaluated the progression of disability in patients with moderate disease from an untreated baseline to an untreated endpoint following medication wash-out over a period of fourteen months [58]. The mean (S.E.) progression in total UPDRS score for selegiline-treated patients was 0.4 (1.3) compared with 5.8 (1.4) in placebo-treated patients (p<0.004). Although it is not possible to be sure that the wash-outs were of sufficient duration, this study is also consistent with the hypothesis that selegiline may slow disease progression.

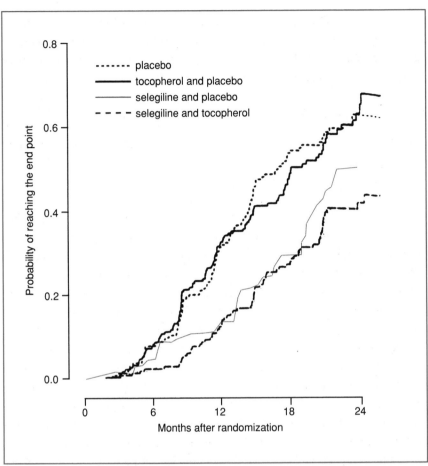

Figure 5-4. *DATATOP results. Kaplan-Meier estimate of the cumulative probability of reaching the end point, according to treatment group. The hazard ratio for patients assigned to selegiline compared to patients assigned to selegiline placebo with respect to the risk of reaching the end point per unit time is 0.50 (p<0.001; 95 percent confidence interval, 0.41 to 0.62).*

Is there any recent information as to how selegiline might provide neuroprotection?

Selegiline appears to afford neuroprotection by mechanisms independent of MAO-B inhibition. Tatton and Greenwood found that selegiline can provide a rescue effect and protect dopaminergic cells in mice from MPTP toxicity even when administered after a delay sufficient to allow the oxidation of MPTP to MPP+ [59]. In cell culture systems, selegiline was found to exert a protective effect by inducing new protein synthesis [60]. Further work suggests that selegiline affects the synthesis of 50 or more proteins and activates a transcriptional program that prevents neurons from entering into apoptosis, a process of cell death [61].

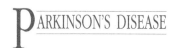

It now appears that one of selegiline's metabolites, desmethylselegiline, is the active molecule for neuroprotection[61]. In contrast, selegiline's amphetamine metabolites may interfere with a neuroprotective effect. Administration of selegiline using a transdermal or nasal formulation avoids first-pass metabolism in the liver and gut, and results in a 60-fold increase in selegiline levels coupled with a 50% reduction in amphetamine metabolites[62]. This suggests that these alternate delivery formulations of selegiline might provide greater neuroprotective effects.

Are there any studies that suggest selegiline may be harmful?

The Parkinson's Disease Research Group of the United Kingdom reported their findings in an open, long-term, prospective trial comparing the effectiveness of levodopa with levodopa combined with selegiline. Five hundred and twenty patients with early Parkinson's disease who were not receiving dopaminergic therapy were randomized to treatment groups and followed for an average of 5.6 years. Disability scores were not significantly different through the observation period. However, they noted 76 deaths in patients assigned to selegiline and levodopa compared to 44 deaths in patients assigned to levodopa alone, representing approximately 57% higher mortality (mortality ratio = 1.57, 95% confidence interval 1.09 to 2.30, log rank test $p = 0.015$)[63]. The difference in mortality emerged between the third and fifth years, and there was no obvious explanation as to the cause of the excess mortality. Differences in mortality were not significant when analyzed for deaths that occurred while patients were still on their assigned treatment (mortality ratio = 1.44, 95% confidence interval = 0.89 to 2.33).

Many questions have been raised regarding the methodology and results of this study including the unusually high mortality rates in both treatment groups (selegiline 28%, non-selegiline 18%), the categorization of the most common cause of death in selegiline-assigned patients as due to "Parkinson's disease", and the apparent lack of appropriate statistical adjustments for interim analyses[62]. It is therefore not clear that the differences between the two groups were statistically significant or that the conclusions of the study are valid. Further, increased mortality has not been identified in any other selegiline study, including DATATOP[64]. Although the report of the Parkinson's Research Group of the United Kingdom raises serious questions, we do not feel this single study warrants a change in selegiline use. The study deserves careful scrutiny and efforts at clarification are required. Extended observations from the DATATOP cohort will also be useful.

What is the role of selegiline in the treatment of Parkinson's disease?

Selegiline delays the need for levodopa in early patients and provides symptomatic benefit for advanced patients with motor fluctuations. In laboratory models, selegiline provides a neuroprotective effect. Although several clinical studies have yielded results which are consistent with a neuroprotective action, this has yet to be conclusively demonstrated in Parkinson's disease patients.

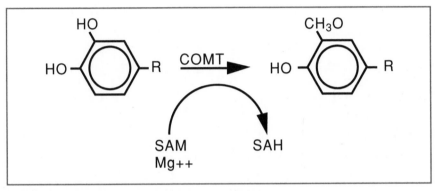

Figure 5-5. *Methylation of catechol substrate by COMT.*
SAM = S-adenosyl-L-methionine; SAH = S-adenosyl-L-homocysteine; R = side chain.

What are COMT inhibitors?

Catechol-O-methyltransferase (COMT) is one of the main enzymes responsible for the metabolism of levodopa, dopamine, other catecholamines (adrenaline and noradrenaline), and their metabolites. COMT catalyzes the transfer of a methyl group from S-adenosyl-L-methionine (SAM) to the hydroxyl group of catecholamines (figure 5-5)[65]. COMT is widely distributed throughout the body [66, 67] including central nervous system neurons and glia, but not nigrostriatal dopamine neurons[68].

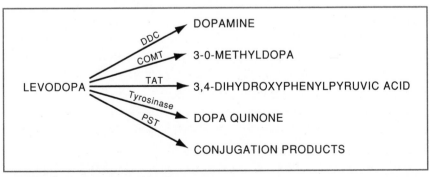

Figure 5-6. *The metabolism of levodopa.*
DDC = dopa decarboxylase; COMT = catechol-O-methyltransferase;
TAT = tyrosine aminotransferase; PST = phenol sulphotransferase.

Levodopa is metabolized by several different enzymes (figure 5-6), with dopa decarboxylase and COMT being most important. When levodopa is administered with a peripheral dopa decarboxylase inhibitor such as carbidopa or benserazide, COMT metabolism of levodopa predominates. COMT metabolizes levodopa to 3-O-methyldopa (3-OMD), a compound which may decrease levodopa absorption and efficacy[69,70]. Peripherally acting COMT inhibitors block COMT in the gut and periphery. By decreasing levodopa metabolism, they make more levodopa available for transport across the blood-brain barrier over a longer time and also reduce 3-OMD production (figure 5-7)[71]. When COMT inhibitors are added to levodopa therapy, striatal dopamine concentrations increase[71]. Central COMT inhibition might further increase striatal dopamine concentration by inhibiting the metabolism of dopamine to homovanillic acid (HVA)[71].

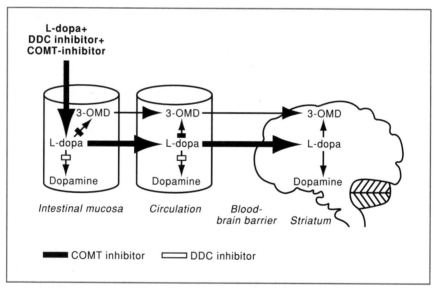

Figure 5-7. *Mechanism of peripheral COMT inhibition.*

What is tolcapone?

Tolcapone is a potent, reversible COMT inhibitor (figure 5-8). Animal studies have demonstrated that tolcapone exerts central as well as peripheral COMT inhibition[71]. It is rapidly absorbed and has a half-life of approximately 2 hours[72]. It is introduced at a dose of 100 or 200 mg TID. Side effects are mostly those relating to increased dopaminergic stimulation[73]. Patients with levodopa-induced dyskinesia often have an initial rapid increase in dyskinesia necessitating a 25-50% reduction in levodopa dose.

Alternatively, the levodopa dose can be reduced by 25-50% at the time tolcapone is initiated and then titrated further as appropriate. Additional dopaminergic side effects include nausea, hallucinations, and hypotension. These side effects can usually be reduced or eliminated by decreasing the levodopa dose. Approximately 10% of patients experience diarrhea and 3% discontinue tolcapone because of this side effect. Onset of diarrhea is usually delayed for four to twelve weeks after initiation of therapy but uncommon after six months[74]. The mechanism of this side effect is unknown.

Tolcapone has been demonstrated in prospective, double-blind studies to improve motor function and allow levodopa dose reductions in patients on levodopa therapy with either a stable response or with motor fluctuations. In a three month study comparing tolcapone (200 mg TID) with placebo in patients with motor fluctuations on levodopa, tolcapone permitted a 24% reduction in levodopa dose compared with a 1.6% increase in placebo-treated patients ($p < .001$)[75]. Mean reduction in "off" time was 18.8% in the tolcapone group compared with 7.8% in the placebo group ($p < .001$). In a six month study evaluating tolcapone in patients on levodopa without motor fluctuations, motor function improved 12% in tolcapone-treated patients compared with 1.5% in placebo-treated patients ($p < .05$ for 100 mg TID, $p < .01$ for 200 mg TID)[74]. Over the six months, placebo patients had a mean increase in levodopa dose of 13% while the tolcapone groups had decreases of 6 and 9% ($p < .001$).

What is entacapone?

Entacapone is a reversible peripheral COMT inhibitor (figure 5-8)[76]. Its half-life is 2 to 3 hours[77] and it is usually administered at a dose of 200 mg with each dose of levodopa. Similar to other COMT inhibitors, most side effects are related to increased dopaminergic stimulation and can be alleviated by reducing the levodopa dose. Entacapone is effective in reducing "off" time and allowing levodopa dose reductions in patients with motor fluctuations on levodopa. In a six month study, motor function had worsened by 9% in the placebo group taking 3% more levodopa than baseline, compared to an improvement in motor function of 1% in the entacapone group taking 13% less levodopa[78]. Entacapone also increased "on" time significantly ($p < .005$).

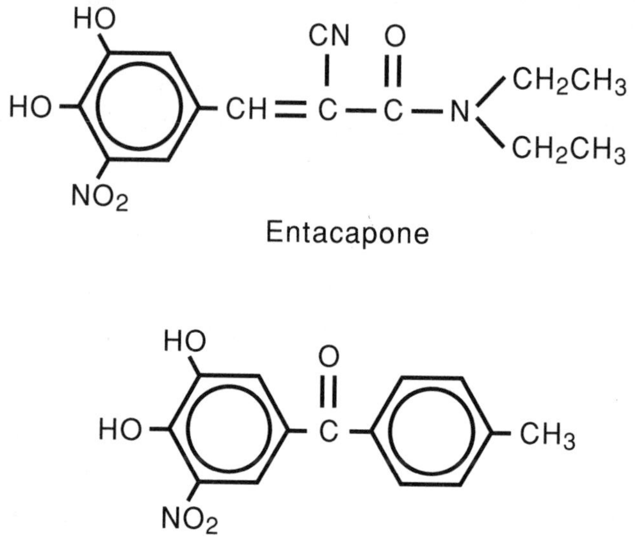

Figure 5-8. *The structures of entacapone and tolcapone.*

What are the "minor" antiparkinsonian medications?

The "minor" antiparkinsonian medications are anticholinergic agents and amantadine. These drugs provide less anti-parkinsonian efficacy than dopaminergic medications.

What are anticholinergic medications?

Anticholinergic medications were the mainstay of anti-parkinsonian treatment until the latter part of this century. They are most effective for reducing tremor[79], and usually provide minimal benefit with regard to bradykinesia and rigidity. In addition, tremor may or may not improve with anticholinergic agents and a given patient may respond to one anticholinergic but not others. Their use is often limited by side effects and they are less well tolerated by older patients and those with dementia. Anticholinergics may cause confusion and hallucinations and most patients experience dry mouth or dry eyes[79]. Additional side effects may include urinary retention, ocular accommodation abnormalities, abnormal sweating, and tachycardia. Anticholinergics should be used with caution in patients with glaucoma.

What are the most frequently used anticholinergic medications?

The most commonly used anticholinergic medications are trihexyphenidyl-HCl, benztropine mesylate, biperiden-HCl, and procyclidine-HCl. Their frequency of use is generally a matter of personal preference.

When are anticholinergic medications useful?

Anticholinergics may be considered for the treatment of tremor that causes functional disability. Patients, caregivers and physicians often focus on tremor because it is so visually obvious. However, most (treatable) disability in Parkinson's disease is due to bradykinesia and rigidity. These signs are best treated with dopaminergic medications, which may or may not improve tremor. Once bradykinesia and rigidity are adequately treated, anticholinergic medication can be considered for the treatment of residual tremor causing functional disability. Some patients with early disease have tremor without bradykinesia or rigidity and these patients may also benefit from anticholinergic therapy.

What is amantadine?

Amantadine, or 1-amino-adamantine is an antiviral medication which was first found to improve symptoms in Parkinson's disease patients while being used to treat Asian influenza in the 1960s. Subsequent trials confirmed that amantadine provides some benefit for the features of Parkinson's disease [80]. Although its exact mechanism of action is unknown, it appears to augment dopamine release, may inhibit dopamine reuptake and may stimulate dopamine receptors [81]. Amantadine is well absorbed and has a long half-life of approximately 24 hours. It is usually administered as 100 mg PO BID or TID. Because of its urinary excretion, it should be used with caution in patients with renal disease. Amantadine is moderately well tolerated, and side effects include hallucinations, confusion, nightmares, ankle edema, dry mouth, and livedo reticularis, an erythematous rash of the lower extremities. Hyponatremia has also been described.

PARKINSON'S DISEASE

CHAPTER 6

COMPLICATIONS OF LONG-TERM THERAPY IN PARKINSON'S DISEASE

What is the usual course of treated Parkinson's disease?

Patients usually experience good control of parkinsonian features when symptomatic therapy is first introduced. This "honeymoon" period is maintained for approximately three to five years into levodopa therapy [1,2]. Although levodopa/PDI has a short serum half-life, patients initially experience a stable response through the day (figure 6-1). This is presumably due to the ability of remaining nigrostriatal neurons to generate dopamine from absorbed levodopa, store it intraneuronally, and slowly release it into the synaptic cleft in a relatively normal fashion. Because there are 60-80% fewer dopamine neurons, the amount of dopamine released from each is increased (increased dopamine turnover) in order to approximate the normal state. Despite levodopa therapy, disability continues to progress [3]. This may be due to inadequate dopamine stimulation or degeneration of neurons downstream to dopamine receptors. Over the years there is a tendency to administer increasing amounts of dopaminergic medication in order to minimize the progression of functional disability.

Between approximately four and eight years, many patients experience motor fluctuations and dyskinesia. Patients begin to notice that whereas they used to be able to take standard levodopa/PDI three or four times a day and still maintain a stable response, the benefit now lasts a few hours and then wears off. Patients may initially notice a short duration levodopa response of four to five hours. Over the next few years, the short duration response becomes more fleeting and benefit lasts only two to three hours. Over time, clinical status more and more closely fluctuates in concert with peripheral levodopa concentration [4]. As neuronal degeneration progresses, the capacity for surviving neurons to effectively store levodopa-derived dopamine diminishes.

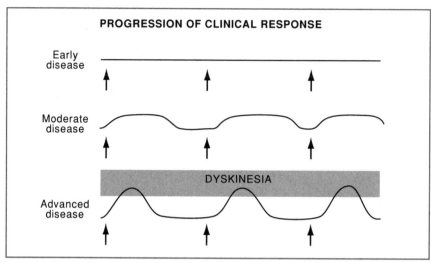

Figure 6-1. *Progression of clinical response in Parkinson's disease. Despite the short half-life of levodopa/PDI, patients with early disease experience a sustained response through the day. As the disease progresses, patients begin to notice "wearing-off" fluctuations such that the benefit of levodopa/PDI wears off after a few hours. Ultimately, clinical response fluctuates more and more closely in association with peripheral levodopa and patients develop choreiform dyskinesia when dopamine peaks. Arrows indicate times of levodopa/PDI administration.*

During this time, many patients also develop peak-dose dyskinesia consisting of choreiform twisting, turning movements that occur when central dopamine levels are peaking [5,6]. This marks an important milestone in the treatment of Parkinson's disease because it limits the amount of dopaminergic therapy that can be provided. At this point, higher doses of dopaminergic therapy are likely to increase peak-dose dyskinesia. This "hypersensitivity" may result from exposing post-synaptic receptors to rapidly fluctuating levodopa-derived dopamine levels [4].

From five to ten years into symptomatic therapy, much of the management of Parkinson's disease centers on titrating therapy to maximize "on" time without dyskinesia. Too much dopaminergic therapy exacerbates peak-dose dyskinesia and too little dopaminergic therapy fails to bring about sufficient benefit. Despite optimal titration, many patients eight or more years into symptomatic therapy suffer with troublesome or disabling motor fluctuations and dyskinesia.

Some patients develop dementia as the disease progresses. As antiparkinsonian therapy can worsen confusion and hallucinations, the presence of cognitive dysfunction can also limit administration of medication to improve motor symptoms.

By ten to twelve years into therapy, many patients have developed balance difficulty. This is another important milestone. True postural imbalance is not improved by any current antiparkinsonian therapy. Patients are then at risk for morbidity and mortality from falls. Immobility may place a patient at increased risk for infections and swallowing difficulty may increase the risk of aspiration and malnutrition.

Individual progression varies greatly. Some patients maintain relatively good function fifteen years into the disease and others experience meaningful disability within a few years.

What are the complications of long-term levodopa therapy in Parkinson's disease?

The complications of long-term therapy for Parkinson's disease include motor fluctuations and dyskinesia. Motor fluctuations consist of variations in clinical status that occur over the course of a day. Dyskinesia refers to abnormal involuntary movements occurring in association with medication therapy.

What are the different types of motor fluctuations?

Wearing-off fluctuations are relatively predictable variations in motor function temporally associated with the timing of levodopa ingestion. After several years of stable response through the day, many patients experience benefit for only a few hours following levodopa ingestion. This is followed by a loss of benefit, or wearing-off. Symptom control can be regained by taking the next levodopa dose. In contrast, on-off fluctuations are rapid transitions (over seconds) between the on and off states, seemingly unrelated to the timing of medication ingestion.

What are the "on" and "off" states?

On and off states can be identified in patients with motor fluctuations. "On" refers to a patient's clinical status when medication is providing symptomatic benefit with regard to mobility, bradykinesia, and rigidity. "Off" refers to a patient's status when symptomatic benefit has been lost over the preceding minutes or hours. Some patients also experience an intermediate state as re-emergence of tremor may precede loss of benefit for mobility, bradykinesia and rigidity.

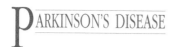

Will my patient recognize motor fluctuations?

Patients with a stable response commonly report that they are unsure if they are experiencing motor fluctuations. In contrast, patients with motor fluctuations can usually identify these fluctuations without difficulty.

Is a worsening of tremor during periods of stress a type of motor fluctuation?

No. Patients commonly experience a transient period of increased tremor (or dyskinesia) when emotionally activated. This phenomenon is not related to the pharmacokinetics of levodopa. Its cause is poorly understood.

What are the types of dyskinesia that occur in Parkinson's disease?

Involuntary abnormal movements associated with medication intake are categorized by the type of movement and the phase of the dosing cycle in which it occurs. The three most common types of dyskinesia in Parkinson's disease are peak-dose dyskinesia, wearing-off dystonia, and diphasic dystonia/dyskinesia. They are relatively specific to Parkinson's disease and often worse on the side of the body most affected . They usually emerge in patients who have had a good response to levodopa and the incidence is highest in young-onset patients [6].

Peak-dose dyskinesias are most common. They occur at the peak of the dosing cycle, when levodopa-derived dopamine is highest. They consist of choreiform, non-patterned, twisting, turning movements usually seen in the extremities, trunk, and head. They diminish when the levodopa dose is reduced and increase when the levodopa dose is raised.

Wearing-off dystonia occurs in association with low or falling dopamine levels [7]. It commonly occurs at night or in the morning prior to the first levodopa dose. It consists of involuntary, sustained muscle contractions and commonly occurs in the lower extremities causing foot inversion or plantar-flexion. The dystonia may be associated with pain, particularly in the calf. It may respond to more sustained dopaminergic stimulation as provided by dopamine agonists or levodopa/carbidopa CR.

Diphasic dystonia/dyskinesia is relatively uncommon and occurs both when a patient is turning on and when he is wearing off. It was originally called D-I-D dystonia, indicating dystonia was followed by improvement and then a return of dystonia within a single dosing cycle [5]. It is often manifest as a combination of dystonia and chorea, and typically affects the lower extremities. Diphasic dyskinesia can be difficult to treat but usually an attempt is made to increase and smooth dopaminergic stimulation.

It can usually be assumed that chorea in the setting of treated Parkinson's disease represents peak-dose dyskinesia until proven otherwise because it is so common. The unqualified term dyskinesia in the context of Parkinson's disease usually refers to peak-dose dyskinesia.

How common are the long-term complications?

More than 50% of patients treated five years or longer may have motor fluctuations and dyskinesia [8].

Are these long-term complications caused by levodopa?

Normal individuals do not appear to develop motor fluctuations or dyskinesia even if taking levodopa. The emergence of long-term complications probably occurs as a result of the combination of disease progression and levodopa administration.

Are dopamine agonists associated with long-term complications?

Motor fluctuations and dyskinesia are uncommon in patients on dopamine agonist monotherapy. Agonists with long half-lives provide a relatively stable clinical response and it is unusual for a patient to experience motor fluctuations on these agents alone. However, patients with advanced disease do experience fluctuations when short-acting dopamine agonists are administered. It is also uncommon for patients to experience dyskinesia on dopamine agonist monotherapy. In contrast, patients with peak-dose dyskinesia on levodopa commonly experience a worsening of dyskinesia when an agonist is added.

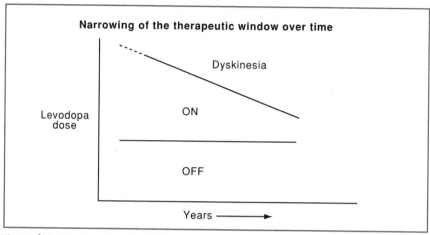

Figure 6-2. *Patients with early Parkinson's disease have a wide therapeutic window and respond well to a wide range of levodopa dosages. As the disease progresses, the therapeutic window narrows. Insufficient dosages in later disease may not bring about benefit (on). High dosages may cause choreiform dyskinesia.*

What is the "therapeutic window"?

Patients with both motor fluctuations and dyskinesia are said to have a therapeutic window. It lies above the threshold required to improve symptoms ("on threshold") and below the threshold for peak-dose dyskinesia ("dyskinesia threshold"). When patients are on without dyskinesia they are said to be in their therapeutic window.

What happens to the therapeutic window over time?

The therapeutic window appears to become smaller over time (figure 6-2). Much of the narrowing of the therapeutic window is due to a progressive lowering of the dyskinesia threshold. Once the window is sufficiently narrowed, it may be difficult to provide much on time without dyskinesia and even optimal medication titration may do no more than provide a balance between off time and dyskinesia.

Which is worse, off time or dyskinesia?

Both off time and dyskinesia can be disabling. Most patients prefer dyskinesia to off time and most family members and physicians prefer for the patient to be off than have dyskinesia. It is important to listen to the patient and help him achieve the balance that he most prefers. Usually the goal is to maximize on time while attempting to minimize troublesome or disabling dyskinesia.

Having the patient fill out a diary divided into half-hour time periods can help the physician analyze the amount of off time and dyskinesia, and their relation to the timing of medication intake (figure 6-3).

What is freezing?

Freezing is a momentary inability to move one's feet during ambulation. Patients will describe that their feet feel stuck to the floor. Start-hesitation is freezing when a patient attempts to initiate ambulation. Freezing generally occurs late in Parkinson's disease and affects roughly one third of patients [9,10]. It occurs more frequently in those whose initial symptoms were gait-related. Freezing may be brought on by turning or attempting to walk through a doorway and may cause or contribute to falls. Response to medication manipulation is usually poor. Tricks or strategies such as attempting to march rather than walk, stepping over an object, or walking over masking tape placed across a walkway may be helpful.

PARKINSON'S DISEASE DIARY

NAME_____   DATE_____

Instructions: For each half-hour time period place one check mark to indicate your predominant status during most of that period.
ON = Time when medication is providing benefit with regard to mobility, slowness, and stiffness.
OFF = Time when medication has worn off and is no longer providing benefit with regard to mobility, slowness, and stiffness.
Dyskinesia = Involuntary twisting, turning movements. These movements are an effect of medication and occur during ON time.
Non-troublesome dyskinesia does not interfere with function or cause meaningful discomfort. **Troublesome dyskinesia** interferes with function or causes meaningful discomfort.
Tremor is shaking back and forth and is not considered dyskinesia.

time	asleep	OFF	ON without dyskinesia	ON with non-troublesome dyskinesia	ON with troublesome dyskinesia	time	asleep	OFF	ON without dyskinesia	ON with non-troublesome dyskinesia	ON with troublesome dyskinesia
6:00 AM						6:00 PM					
:30						:30					
7:00 AM						7:00 PM					
:30						:30					
8:00 AM						8:00 PM					
:30						:30					
9:00 AM						9:00 PM					
:30						:30					
10:00 AM						10:00 PM					
:30						:30					
11:00 AM						11:00 PM					
:30						:30					
12:00 PM						12:00 AM					
:30						:30					
1:00 PM						1:00 AM					
:30						:30					
2:00 PM						2:00 AM					
:30						:30					
3:00 PM						3:00 AM					
:30						:30					
4:00 PM						4:00 AM					
:30						:30					
5:00 PM						5:00 AM					
:30						:30					

Figure 6-3. *Parkinson's disease diary.*

PARKINSON'S DISEASE

CHAPTER 7

MEDICAL MANAGEMENT OF PARKINSON'S DISEASE

What is the goal of medical management of Parkinson's disease?

The goal of medical management of Parkinson's disease is to adequately control signs and symptoms while minimizing side effects for as long as possible.

What are some general guidelines for the use of medications in Parkinson's disease?

We prefer to make only one medication change at a time so that the positive and negative effects of that change are clear.

We institute symptomatic medications at a low dose and slowly escalate based on clinical response in order to minimize the incidence of early side effects. Signs and symptoms progress slowly and rapid medication changes are rarely required.

Although knowledge and experience are useful guides, each patient must be assessed and treated as an individual.

Will medications eliminate the signs and symptoms of Parkinson's disease?

Except in very early disease, medications will not entirely eliminate signs and symptoms of Parkinson's disease. As the disease progresses, symptoms increase despite best medical management. Asymmetry often persists with worse signs apparent in the first-affected extremity.

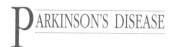

How do I know if an increase in medication is warranted?

The presence of functional disability warrants a trial of increased medication. Experience is the best guide to realistic expectations. Nonetheless, if symptom control is inadequate, an attempt to bring about improvement is warranted. If no improvement can be achieved before intolerable side effects emerge, the lowest medication dose that will maintain the current level of function is appropriate.

What is your general approach to the medical treatment of Parkinson's disease?

We attempt to provide adequate symptomatic control throughout the course of the disease. The younger and healthier the patient, the more aggressively we base our treatment on strategies designed to maximize function over the long term. This includes the use of dopamine agonist monotherapy as part of a strategy to spare levodopa and provide smooth dopamine receptor stimulation. This approach can be easily implemented without compromising symptomatic control.

When do you introduce symptomatic medication therapy for Parkinson's disease?

Symptomatic medications are initiated when the patient begins to experience functional disability. Patients with early disease should be monitored clinically for the development of functional disability.

What is functional disability?

Functional disability is present when symptoms of Parkinson's disease interfere with activities the patient either wants or needs to do. This should be assessed individually for each patient in the context of his lifestyle. A small loss of finger dexterity may threaten a keyboard operator's livelihood and warrant symptomatic therapy, whereas a retiree may have greater motor dysfunction without disability and may not require symptomatic therapy.

What should I do when a patient develops functional disability?

Symptomatic therapy should be initiated when functional disability emerges. For most patients we prefer to begin symptomatic therapy with a dopamine agonist. Dopamine agonists provide anti-parkinsonian benefit approximately equal to levodopa therapy for six months to a year and may adequately control symptoms for several years. Levodopa is added when agonist therapy no longer provides sufficient symptomatic benefit. By starting symptomatic therapy with a dopamine agonist we delay the need for levodopa and provide relatively smooth dopamine receptor stimulation. Once levodopa therapy becomes necessary, we are able to use lower doses when it is administered concurrently with an agonist. There is increasing evidence to suggest that this approach may be associated with a lower prevalence of dyskinesia [1-3].

For elderly patients and those with dementia, we place less emphasis on long-term considerations and may elect to use levodopa as the first symptomatic agent. We use the lowest levodopa dosage that will adequately control symptoms. We may also elect to use levodopa as the first symptomatic agent for patients who are very immobile, bradykinetic or rigid, and for those in whom we need to bring about rapid improvement. A dopamine agonist can then be introduced shortly thereafter when reasonable control of parkinsonian symptoms has been achieved.

How do you dose the dopamine agonists?

The agonists are best introduced at a low dose and slowly escalated. Reasonably high doses should be achieved before their utility is assessed. An opportunity for improvement may be lost if they are judged ineffective at low doses.

What should I do when dopamine agonist therapy no longer provides adequate symptomatic control?

Levodopa therapy is required when dopamine agonists no longer provide adequate symptomatic control. We favor continuing the agonist and adding levodopa. This may reduce the long-term incidence of motor complications [2,3]. In addition, less levodopa is required, levodopa-induced free radical formation may be diminished, and dopamine receptors are buffered from fluctuating concentrations of levodopa-derived dopamine.

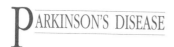

What is the role of COMT inhibitors?

COMT inhibitors can improve motor function in patients with a stable response to levodopa/PDI, and can reduce off time and improve motor function in patients with motor fluctuations. They extend the peripheral half-life of levodopa and increase its bio-availability. COMT inhibitors are very helpful to reduce off time in patients with motor fluctuations. In addition, COMT inhibitors can be added to the antiparkinsonian regimen when the response to a low dose of levodopa/PDI (~ 400 mg.) is waning, as an alternative to increasing the levodopa dose. The strategy of smoothing dopamine receptor stimulation can be maximized with the concurrent administration of a COMT inhibitor and a dopamine agonist as adjuncts to levodopa, thereby providing a rationale for the introduction of a COMT inhibitor at the time levodopa therapy is begun.

What levodopa formulation should I use when levodopa therapy is first required?

We favor using a controlled-release levodopa preparation when levodopa therapy is first required. It provides as much symptomatic benefit as standard levodopa and can be dosed less frequently. In addition, there is interest in whether the smoother receptor stimulation afforded by controlled-release levodopa in comparison to standard levodopa can forestall the development of fluctuations and dyskinesia. A recent 5-year study found greater improvement in Activities of Daily Living scores in patients randomized to CR levodopa/carbidopa than standard levodopa/carbidopa although the incidence of fluctuations and dyskinesia was similar in both groups[4].

How do I dose levodopa?

It is helpful to introduce levodopa at a low dose and then escalate slowly to minimize the incidence of side effects. We introduce carbidopa/levodopa CR at a dose of one 25/100 tablet per day and escalate to a target dose of 25/100 TID over one month. We introduce standard carbidopa/levodopa at a dose of one half of a 25/100 tablet per day and escalate to a target of either one half tablet QID or one tablet TID over one month. Further escalations are undertaken based on clinical response.

What is the usual timeline for this long-term strategy?

There is a lot of variability in the rate of progression of Parkinson's disease. Nonetheless, most patients will require symptomatic therapy within one to two years of diagnosis. Once functional disability emerges, a dopamine agonist will often control symptoms for another one to three years.

How much levodopa is too much?

Most experts try to keep the levodopa dose below 500 - 600 mg per day for as long as possible. Despite this, patients should receive as much levodopa as is necessary to adequately control symptoms. If the patient has sufficient bradykinesia and rigidity to cause meaningful disability, the levodopa dose should be increased. There is no maximal levodopa dose, and some patients require relatively high doses (~1000 - 1500 mg levodopa/PDI or more) to achieve good benefit. At some point in a levodopa escalation, the patient will encounter an intolerable side effect and this defines "too much" levodopa for that patient. If the levodopa dose is escalated and no additional benefit occurs, the dose should be tapered down to the lowest dose that still provides the current level of benefit. Higher levodopa dosages that do not bring about additional benefit should be avoided.

What does it mean if there is no improvement when I add levodopa?

Almost all Parkinson's disease patients with sufficient bradykinesia and rigidity will experience improvement when levodopa therapy is introduced. There are several reasons why there may be no appreciable response. The dose may be too low, the diagnosis may be wrong, attention may be focused on the wrong symptoms, or symptoms may be so slight that improvement is hard to identify. Most Parkinson's disease patients experience noticeable improvement with 600 mg of levodopa/PDI per day or less. Much of this improvement is reduced bradykinesia and rigidity, and increased mobility and dexterity. If no improvement is noted, and symptoms remain prominent, the dose should be slowly escalated to tolerance. Improvement in bradykinesia and rigidity may be overlooked if too much attention is focused on tremor. Tremor may or may not respond to levodopa. If the patient has minimal difficulty with bradykinesia, rigidity, dexterity and mobility, improvement may be hard to detect. Normal individuals and patients with atypical parkinsonism usually do not benefit from levodopa therapy.

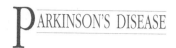

Patients who have been on levodopa for some time may be unaware of the benefit that it is providing. If there is a question as to whether levodopa is providing benefit, a temporary taper is often helpful.

How should I approach the treatment of tremor?

Tremor usually does not cause much functional disability in Parkinson's disease. We attempt to treat bradykinesia and rigidity with dopaminergic medications and then evaluate residual tremor. If a functionally disabling tremor persists or is the only manifestation of Parkinson's disease, we introduce an anticholinergic medication. Tremor is variably responsive to levodopa, dopamine agonists and anticholinergic medications. In addition, tremor may respond to one anticholinergic but not another, so it is worth trying several (sequentially) if necessary. Patients with medically refractory, disabling tremor may benefit from a surgical procedure such as thalamotomy or chronic thalamic stimulation.

What if my patient can't tolerate levodopa/PDI?

The long-term treatment of Parkinson's disease without levodopa is almost always less than satisfactory. When a patient has disabling parkinsonian symptoms it is very important to employ all conceivable strategies to try to achieve tolerability. Smaller doses than were previously used should be employed to reintroduce the medication. If necessary, a standard levodopa tablet can be crushed and one small chip per day used as the starting dose. If a patient has difficulty initiating levodopa therapy due to nausea, he should be instructed to take it immediately following a meal. If nausea persists, additional carbidopa or benserazide may be helpful. Carbidopa is available directly from the manufacturer. Although 80 mg of carbidopa per day is usually sufficient to saturate peripheral decarboxylase, some patients will benefit from carbidopa in doses up to 200 mg per day. In some cases, a peripheral dopamine blocker such as domperidone will be required, and this is usually quite effective. For patients whose intolerability is due to orthostatic hypotension, fludrocortisone or midodrine may be beneficial.

How can I treat motor fluctuations?

After several years of a stable response through the day, many patients on levodopa begin to experience motor fluctuations and notice that the benefit wears off after a few hours. It is usually relatively easy to reduce off time in a patient with motor fluctuations who is not experiencing peak-dose dyskinesia. Several different strategies, alone or in combination, can be used to provide more sustained dopaminergic therapy. Possible strategies include adding selegiline, a dopamine agonist, or a COMT inhibitor, dosing levodopa more frequently, increasing the levodopa dose, or switching from standard to a long-acting preparation (figure 7-1). The patient should be alerted to the fact that increased dopaminergic therapy may cause or worsen peak-dose dyskinesia.

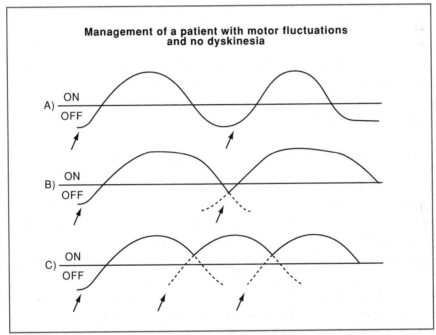

Figure 7-1. *Management of a patient with motor fluctuations and no dyskinesia (A). Off time can be reduced by using a higher levodopa dose (B), switching to a long acting preparation (B), adding a dopamine agonist, COMT inhibitor or selegiline (B), or by shortening the interdose interval (C). Arrows indicate times of levodopa administration.*

How do I manage patients with both motor fluctuations and dyskinesia?

Patients with both motor fluctuations and troublesome peak-dose dyskinesia can present a difficult management challenge. The goal of treatment for these patients is to provide as much good functional time through the day as possible. This is accomplished by maximizing on time without dyskinesia and on time with non-troublesome (mild) dyskinesia. An attempt is made to reduce both off time and troublesome or disabling dyskinesia. An increase in dopaminergic therapy may increase dyskinesia and a decrease in dopaminergic therapy may increase off time. For many patients with severe fluctuations and dyskinesia, the best that can be done is to balance off time and dyskinesia. The patient's relative preference for off time versus dyskinesia should be taken into account.

Improvement is sought by attempting to provide as stable dopaminergic stimulation as possible within the therapeutic target zone. The addition of selegiline, a dopamine agonist, or a COMT inhibitor may be helpful. Dyskinesia may increase when these medications are added and downward titration of levodopa should then be undertaken. For patients on controlled-release levodopa it is often helpful to switch to a standard levodopa/PDI preparation to provide a more consistent and predictable dosing cycle (figure 7-2). It is then critical to titrate the dose based on clinical response. In general, it is desirable to administer smaller levodopa doses more frequently. A dose should be sought which is sufficient to turn the patient on without causing too much dyskinesia (figure 7-3). The time to wearing-off then determines the appropriate interdose interval. Ideally, the next dose should be given to take effect when the previous dose begins to wear off. In advanced disease, if a patient's response has become extremely erratic, he may have to take his next dose when he feels the previous dose wearing off rather than adhering to a fixed dosing schedule.

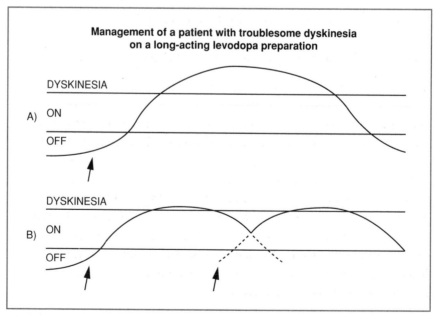

Figure 7-2. *Patients with troublesome dyskinesia while on a long-acting levodopa preparation (A) may benefit from a switch to standard levodopa/PDI (B). This may allow for better titration and a more consistent dosing cycle. Arrows indicate times of levodopa administration.*

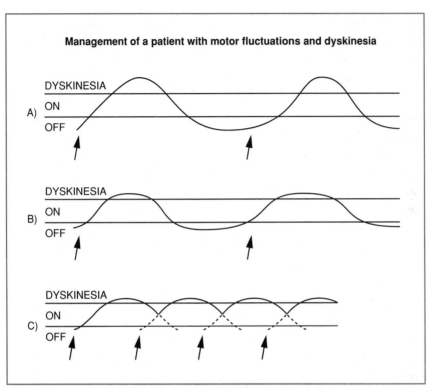

Figure 7-3. *The treatment of patients with motor fluctuations and peak-dose dyskinesia (A) generally involves providing less levodopa more frequently. The levodopa dose should be lowered until it brings on only mild dyskinesia (B). The time to wearing off then determines the interdose interval (C). Arrows indicate times of levodopa administration.*

Does diet play a role in motor fluctuations?

Levodopa competes with other large neutral amino acids for transport across the blood-brain barrier. Protein ingested in meals can slow levodopa flow into the brain. This usually has no impact on patients with relatively early disease, but can have a dramatic effect on patients with more advanced disease as clinical status becomes critically dependent on continuous levodopa transport into the brain. Patients with severe fluctuations and those who find they turn off following a meal may benefit from a low protein or protein redistributed diet[5]. In addition, balanced carbohydrate-protein commercial food preparations are available. For patients with severe motor fluctuations, minimizing serum protein fluctuations may reduce the variability of levodopa transport and help provide a more stable clinical response.

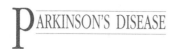

How can I make levodopa take effect faster?

For patients with motor fluctuations, levodopa/PDI commonly takes 20-30 minutes or more before an effect is apparent. By chewing the tablet, the absorption rate is increased and clinical benefit occurs more rapidly. This may be particularly useful for patients taking levodopa on an as needed basis when the previous dose has worn off and for patients who awaken immobile at night and need symptomatic benefit as quickly as possible.

How can I manage my patients with severe fluctuations and dyskinesia?

Patients with severe fluctuations and dyskinesia often gain some benefit when placed on a "liquid levodopa" regimen[6]. Patients are instructed to dissolve ten standard carbidopa/levodopa 25/100 tablets in one liter of water with one-half teaspoon of ascorbic acid. The result is a one mg per milliliter levodopa solution. The solution should be made fresh every day and hourly dosing is usually employed. An initial dosing schedule is calculated and further adjustments must be made to titrate to clinical response.

The first dose of the day is the same as had been taken in pill form. Initial hourly doses are calculated by dividing the patient's prior daily levodopa dose by the number of hourly doses he will be taking. When possible, the first daily dose is adjusted before the hourly doses. Adjustments are made in 5 mg increments every three to five days. Rather precise measurements are required for consistent dosing and most of our patients use a 60 cc syringe to measure each dose. For successful initiation of liquid therapy it is critical to inform patients that the initial recommended schedule is only a rough guess as to dosing.

The ultimate benefit of a liquid regimen can only be assessed after optimal titration which usually takes several weeks. Without this warning patients are likely to abandon liquid therapy in the first few days when they experience increased off time or dyskinesia. Aggressive titration is vital. Most patients on liquid therapy use the levodopa solution through the day and take a CR tablet at bedtime to help them get through the night.

How do I treat wearing-off dystonia?

Wearing-off dystonia often responds to more sustained dopaminergic therapy. Substantial improvement is usually brought about by the addition of a dopamine agonist. Some patients benefit from a bedtime dose of a long acting levodopa preparation.

How do I treat diphasic dyskinesia?

Diphasic dyskinesia can be difficult to treat. In general, an attempt is made to increase and smooth dopaminergic stimulation. The goal is to avoid turning on and wearing-off as much as possible since these are the phases of the dosing cycle in which diphasic dyskinesia occurs.

What should I do if my patient is confused?

Dementia occurs in approximately 15-30% of Parkinson's disease patients[7]. It typically occurs late in the disease and progresses over time. Confusion can be exacerbated by medications. If confusion is present a review of all of the patient's medications is in order to identify those that are particularly associated with confusion. Any unnecessary medications should be discontinued. Any of the anti-parkinsonian medications can cause or exacerbate confusion. If confusion is evident, anti-parkinsonian medications should be reduced to see if improvement can be achieved. We first reduce and eliminate the minor anti-parkinsonian medications including amantadine and the anticholinergics. We may then reduce and eliminate the dopamine agonists. If necessary, the levodopa dose is reduced. In some cases the best balance between motor control and confusion must be sought using levodopa/PDI alone.

What should I do if my patient experiences hallucinations?

One must evaluate the impact of hallucinations on the patient. If they are mild and non-bothersome, no change may be necessary. An attempt should be made to alleviate more severe hallucinations. The minor anti-parkinsonian medications, and if necessary, the dopamine agonists can be discontinued. The levodopa dose can be decreased to see if hallucinations can be ameliorated while still maintaining control of motor symptoms.

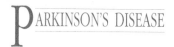

If a satisfactory balance between motor symptom control and hallucinations cannot be achieved by titrating levodopa, consideration is given to adding an atypical neuroleptic. Classical neuroleptics such as haloperidol may reduce hallucinations but are likely to worsen motor symptoms. The preferred treatment is clozapine, an atypical neuroleptic with minimal parkinsonian side effects [8]. The most common side effect of clozapine is hypotension. The main serious side effect is the risk of neutropenia. Because of this risk, weekly monitoring of the patient's white blood cell count is required. Clozapine is quite effective in reducing hallucinations but does not improve underlying dementia. The doses used to treat hallucinations in Parkinson's disease are much lower than those used to treat schizophrenia. We initiate therapy with a chip (~ one-eighth) of a 25 mg tablet and slowly escalate to one quarter tablet the second week and one half tablet the third week. Most patients require a daily dose of 25 mg or less. Resperidone is another atypical neuroleptic that is effective in reducing hallucinations but it has more parkinsonian side effect than clozapine.

How can I treat Atypical Parkinsonism?

Anti-parkinsonian medications usually do not provide meaningful benefit for the clinical features of Atypical Parkinsonisms. Nonetheless, we usually perform a levodopa trial, introducing it at a low dose and slowly escalating until intolerable side effects emerge. We hope to achieve a levodopa dose of approximately 1000 - 1500 mg to be satisfied that an adequate trial has been completed. If no benefit is realized, we taper the dose downward to see if a loss of symptomatic benefit can be identified. When benefit occurs it is usually modest and fleeting. Medication is discontinued if no benefit is identified. One of the reasons we perform a levodopa trial is to be sure we have not misdiagnosed an unusual presentation of Parkinson's disease and missed an opportunity for improvement. Much of the management of Atypical Parkinsonisms is supportive. Secondary symptoms such as depression and constipation should be aggressively sought and treated.

CHAPTER 8

MANAGEMENT OF SECONDARY SYMPTOMS OF PARKINSON'S DISEASE

How should I approach depression in Parkinson's disease?

Depression is the most common mood disturbance in Parkinson's disease, affecting roughly 40 to 50% of patients[1]. Parkinson's disease patients experience major depression more frequently than the normal elderly, and are significantly more depressed than nonparkinsonian control patients with comparable disability[2]. Depressed Parkinson's disease patients often meet clinical criteria for either major depression or dysthymic disorder[2,3] and often have concurrent symptoms of panic and anxiety[4]. Most studies have not found an association between depression in Parkinson's disease and severity or duration of illness, age, or gender[5]. In general, Parkinson's disease patients have less self-blame and guilt than their depressed, nonparkinsonian counterparts[6].

It is unclear whether the etiology of depression in Parkinson's disease is endogenous, reactive, or both. There is evidence that depression in Parkinson's disease is related to serotonergic abnormalities[7]. Nonetheless, it appears likely that both neurochemical changes and psychosocial issues may contribute to the development of depression in Parkinson's disease.

Antidepressants have been found to improve depression in Parkinson's disease patients in a limited number of studies[8-10]. Tricyclic antidepressants, serotonin reuptake inhibitors, and atypical antidepressants have all been found to improve depression in Parkinson's disease patients. However, several case reports have noted worsening of parkinsonian symptoms after treatment with the serotonin reuptake inhibitors fluoxetine and paroxetine[11,12]. An open label study of sertraline found it to reduce depression in stable Parkinson's disease patients without worsening motor symptoms[13].

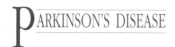
What is the serotonin syndrome?

Selective serotonin reuptake inhibitors (SSRI's) are commonly used to treat depression in Parkinson's disease. However, SSRI's, either alone or in combination with monoamine oxidase inhibitors such as selegiline, can cause the "serotonin syndrome", characterized by mental status changes, tremor, diaphoresis, and incoordination. Deaths have occurred due to rhabdomyolysis, disseminated intravascular coagulation, respiratory distress syndrome, and cardiovascular collapse [14-16]. Treatment of the serotonin syndrome involves discontinuation of the inciting drug and supportive measures, with resolution of symptoms usually occurring in hours to weeks [17].

The occurence of serotonin syndrome in Parkinson's disease patients receiving both selegiline and SSRI's is rare. A retrospective chart review evaluating the concomitant use of fluoxetine and selegiline failed to uncover any serious side effects or additional adverse events which had not already been reported with each medication alone [18].

How do I treat orthostatic hypotension?

Orthostatic hypotension is defined as a drop of 30 mm Hg in systolic blood pressure or a drop of 20 mm Hg in mean blood pressure (diastolic plus one third of the pulse pressure) when going from the supine to standing position. Asymptomatic orthostatic hypotension does not require intervention but patients whose blood pressure is no higher than 80/50 mm Hg are usually symptomatic. Associated symptoms include syncope and presyncope but they may also be non-specific such as fatigue, unsteadiness, or cognitive slowing, especially in the elderly.

As a first step, unnecessary medications should be discontinued. The patient should drink five or more glasses of fluid each day and liberally add salt (up to 150-250 mEq) to the diet. Pharmacologic treatment can be undertaken to increase intravascular volume with mineralocorticoids [19], or to increase vascular resistance through stimulation of alpha receptors [20,21]. The mineralocorticoid fludrocortisone is introduced at a dose of 0.1 mg once or twice a day and can be increased to as high as 0.4 to 0.6 mg per day. Supine hypertension and dependent edema are common and not unexpected but care must be taken to avoid congestive heart failure.

Midodrine is a peripherally acting alpha-1-agonist that produces vasoconstriction of both arterioles and venous capacitance vessels [22,23]. The initial recommended dosage is 2.5 mg BID or TID. The usual maintenance dose is 30 mg/day in divided doses, with a maximum of 40 mg/day. It is well absorbed orally and generally well tolerated. Side effects include scalp pruritus and tingling, pilomotor reactions, gastrointestinal complaints, headache, and dizziness [22]. Because it does not cross the blood-brain barrier, it is less likely to produce central nervous system side effects than ephedrine [24]. As a selective alpha-adrenergic agonist, it is relatively free of beta-adrenergic side effects and pulse rate usually does not increase [22]. Patients with supine hypertension (>150/90) should be treated by elevating the head of the bed to a 30 degree incline. Several open label and double-blind studies have shown that midodrine effectively controls symptoms of orthostatic hypotension in most patients [20,25]. Refractory cases may respond to combination therapy with fludrocortisone and midodrine [20].

What is the treatment of constipation in Parkinson's disease?

Constipation is common in Parkinson's disease. In a study comparing colonic transit time between Parkinson's disease patients and age and sex-matched controls, Parkinson's disease patients had delayed colonic transit affecting all segments of the colon [26]. Additional studies have identified decreased basal anal sphincter pressures and a hyper-contractile external sphincter response [27-29].

Colonic abnormalities in Parkinson's disease may have both central and peripheral causes. Lewy bodies have been found in the myenteric plexus of the colon, suggesting that Parkinson's disease may affect the enteric nervous system. There is also a report of the presence of Lewy bodies in the neurons of the dorsal group of the nucleus intermediolateralis of the 3rd sacral segment of the spinal cord [30]. Anismus, or paradoxical contraction of the striated sphincter muscles during defecation, may be part of a focal dystonia. Administration of apomorphine has resulted in improved defecation, suggesting that these problems may be related to dopamine deficiency [31].

Basic treatment of constipation is aimed at increasing stool bulk by adding more fiber to the diet and by increasing daily liquid intake. Fiber intake can be increased by having the patient eat more fruits and raw vegetables,

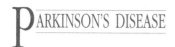

as well as products containing bran. Exercise may also be helpful in alleviating constipation. Anticholinergics which inhibit gastric motility and promote GI dryness should be discontinued. Despite these measures, many patients still complain of significant straining and hard stools. Stool softeners such as docusate sodium may be necessary.

An extremely useful medication is the gastrointestinal prokinetic agent cisapride [32]. Cisapride increases gastric motility by enhancing acetylcholine release at the myenteric plexus. It does not induce muscarinic or nicotinic stimluation. Clinical studies have confirmed reduced colonic transit times with the addition of cisapride [33]. Cisapride has been shown to increase peak plasma levels of levodopa by accelerating gastric emptying and it may have some utility as an add-on medication in the treatment of Parkinson's disease [34]. For patients with refractory constipation, lactulose preparations may be required. When possible, the long term use of pharmacologic agents in treating constipation should be avoided. The simplest measures are best tolerated long-term.

How can I treat drooling?

It is estimated that 70% of Parkinson's disease patients eventually experience drooling [35]. Siallorhea in Parkinson's disease is probably caused by saliva pooling in the mouth secondary to swallowing difficulties, rather than from increased production of saliva [36]. Besides being bothersome to the patient, siallorhea can lead to more serious problems including chemical dermatitis or aspiration. For some patients, increased dopaminergic therapy is useful to improve swallowing and reduce drooling. Anticholinergic medications can reduce saliva production, but may cause side effects including dry mouth, constipation, and cognitive changes. The peripheral anticholinergic glycopyrrolate may be particularly useful to avoid cognitive side effects. For the most difficult cases, salivary duct sclerosis may be considered.

How can I treat dysphagia?

Dysphagia is also common in Parkinson's disease and patients often describe a "choking" sensation along with difficulty swallowing foods. Parkinson's disease can cause esophageal dysfunction and abnormalities in the oropharyngeal phase of swallowing. In one study of swallowing disorders in asymptomatic elderly patients with Parkinson's disease, videofluoroscopy was performed to evaluate facial, tongue, and palatopharyngeal musculature[37]. Although these patients denied any dysphagic symptoms, all patients had at least one abnormality of the swallowing mechanism. Oropharyngeal transit time was increased and patients needed more swallows to remove the bolus from the pharynx. Lewy bodies have been found in the myenteric plexus in the esophagus in dysphagic Parkinson's disease patients[38], again suggesting that the enteric nervous system is affected. Radionucleotide motility studies have revealed slow transit time and demonstrated that dysphagia may improve with medication[39]. Dysphagia may increase the risk of aspiration, although one study failed to demonstrate increased rates of pulmonary infection in Parkinson's disease patients with dysphagia[40].

Parkinson's disease patients with dysphagia should eliminate hard foods from the diet and pay careful attention to swallowing. Increased dopaminergic therapy with levodopa may improve swallowing[41]. For patients with clinically significant dysphagia it is worthwhile to slowly increase the levodopa dose to tolerance to evaluate whether any improvement in dysphagia can be achieved.

How should I approach urinary incontinence in Parkinson's disease?

Patients complaining of urinary symptoms should have a urologic evaluation including cystometric studies to exclude other causes of urinary symptoms, including prostate abnormalities. Decreased levels of dopamine can cause detrusor hyperreflexia in Parkinson's disease patients, resulting in urinary frequency, urgency, and most commonly nocturia. A high incidence of instability of the detrusor muscles has been reported in incontinent Parkinson's disease patients[42].

A simple reduction in fluids after dinner may help to reduce nocturia[42]. Otherwise, use of an anticholinergic medication such as oxybutinin or propantheline may be helpful. Oxybutinin is given in dosages of 5 to 10 mg at bedtime, and propantheline is administered in dosages of 15 to 30 mg at bedtime. Patients should be monitored for cognitive side effects. If detrusor hypoactivity is present, a reduction in anticholinergic medications may be warranted. The use of desmopressin nasal spray to treat nocturia in Parkinson's disease has recently been explored. It may be considered for patients with significant adverse impact due to nocturia refractory to other measures[43].

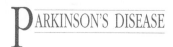

How should I approach sexual dysfunction in Parkinson's disease?

Sexual dysfunction can occur for a variety of reasons including lack of mobility, loss of interest, or difficulty achieving and maintaining erection. Nonetheless, the exact pathophysiology of sexual dysfunction is largely unknown. Loss of sexual interest is commonly reported in Parkinson's disease patients, and both men and women are affected. However, one study suggested that loss of sexual interest, although common, is no greater than that which occurs in other non-neurologic chronic diseases[44]. Depression and use of medications such as propranolol and other antihypertensives can contribute to sexual dysfunction[45,46]. After discontinuation of potentially offending medications and treatment of depression, a patient complaining of sexual dysfunction should be evaluated by a urologist to exclude other causes and direct further management. The use of an externally applied device during sexual intercourse can help men achieve and maintain an erection.

How should I treat seborrhea?

It is not uncommon to find excessive oiliness of the skin, particularly of the forehead, in Parkinson's disease patients. If clinically warranted, the use of topical steroids may be beneficial. If there is an inadequate response, referral to a dermatologist for further evaluation and treatment is appropriate.

How can I treat postural instability (imbalance)?

There is no medication therapy that is known to be effective to treat true balance dysfunction. However, there are multiple reasons why a patient with Parkinson's disease may be prone to falls. If a patient is falling because of poor mobility or shortened gait, improvement may occur with increased levodopa therapy. In addition, the patient's neurologic status should be carefully reviewed to determine if any non-Parkinson's disease signs are contributing to falls. This might include sensory dysfunction that might be amenable to treatment, and weakness that might be the result of stroke or other neurologic disorders.

In general, the approach to postural instability is to try to keep the patient active but safe. Some patients benefit from the use of a three-wheeled walker with hand brakes, and some may benefit from physical therapy. Unfortunately, these are only temporizing measures as postural instability is likely to progress once present.

What role does rehabilitation play in the treatment of Parkinson's disease?

Motor disability in Parkinson's disease may lead to disuse atrophy and contractures. Rehabilitative efforts are often aimed at improving motor function, increasing range of motion, and building endurance. Physical therapy programs generally include therapeutic exercises, gait training, and psychosocial support.

There have been limited evaluations of rehabilitation therapy for Parkinson's disease patients. One open label study identified improvement in strength, initiation of movement, range of motion, and relaxation following a regimen of gymnasium activities [47]. Another study noted improved mobility, feeding, and self care following a home exercise regimen [48]. In the most rigorous study to date, Comella et al. conducted a single-blind, randomized, crossover trial evaluating physical disability after 4 weeks of normal activity and 4 weeks of intensive physical rehabilitation [49]. Significant improvement in UPDRS, ADL, and motor scores were documented following rehabilitation, but scores returned to baseline after six months. Most patients returned to a sedentary lifestyle after structured rehabilitation was completed. This emphasizes the need for long-term maintenance physical activity programs.

PARKINSON'S DISEASE

CHAPTER 9

SURGERY FOR PARKINSON'S DISEASE

Why is there a resurgence of interest in surgical procedures for Parkinson's disease?

The limitations of medical therapy are the driving force behind the development of surgical procedures for the treatment of Parkinson's disease. Surgical procedures were relatively common in the 1950s as adequate medical therapy was not available. With the introduction of levodopa, the perceived need for surgical therapies was greatly reduced and few procedures were performed in the late 1960s and through the 1970s. By the 1980s, the long term inadequacies of levodopa therapy were apparent. In addition, increased understanding of the neuroanatomic pathophysiology of Parkinson's disease allowed rational targets for surgical procedures to be identified. Advances in brain imaging and electrophysiologic recording provided hope that these targets could be accessed with greater precision and consistency. Improved stereotactic surgical techniques lowered morbidity and mortality. The convergence of these advances rekindled interest in surgical procedures. In the 1980's many of the earlier procedures were re-evaluated and new ones introduced.

What types of surgery are being evaluated?

The three basic types of surgery for Parkinson's disease are lesioning, stimulation, and implantation. Lesioning involves the destruction of a target site to modify function. Most lesions today are created by the application of electrothermal energy. Stimulation procedures involve the implantation of an electrode with an exposed tip into a target site. The electrode is connected to a wire run beneath the skin to a stimulator placed in the chest wall. When electrical current is activated it modifies the function of the target site. The principal advantage of stimulation is that it provides a degree of control. The stimulator can be adjusted externally using a programmer with an electromagnetic head. If a side effect occurs due to

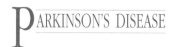

electrical stimulation, the stimulation can be reduced and the side effect will resolve. Implantation involves the delivery of tissue or other material into a target site. It is hoped that implanted cells can replace lost neurons to restore function. The delivery of materials such as growth factors might protect vulnerable neurons from further degeneration.

What were the first surgeries attempted for Parkinson's disease?

Pollack and Davis initially performed posterior rhizotomies (cutting sensory nerve roots as they enter the spinal cord) to reduce rigidity in Parkinson's disease[1]. Although rigidity was improved, tremor was unchanged and sensory loss and contracture formation were problematic. Attention then turned to lesioning the corticospinal motor tracts. Bucy undertook subpial excision of Brodman's cortical area 4[2]. This improved tremor but caused contralateral hemiparesis. Putnam performed cervical pyramidotomy reasoning that lesioning the spinal cord would be associated with a lower incidence of seizures[3]. This procedure induced transient contralateral hemiparesis and transient resolution of tremor. Tremor returned as motor function recovered. Walker later sectioned the lateral two thirds of the cerebral peduncle to induce partial paralysis and incomplete tremor control[4]. It soon became apparent that lesions of the corticospinal system alleviated tremor only at the cost of motor weakness and other features of Parkinson's disease were not improved[5]. Lesioning procedures were then directed to the extrapyramidal system.

What is the history of surgery of the basal ganglia to treat Parkinson's disease?

Myers used a transventricular approach to lesion the caudate and anterior limit of the internal capsule, and to divide the ansa lenticularis which contains the major outflow form the pallidum to the thalamus[6,7]. Tremor was reduced in more than 60% of patients but the procedure was associated with a 12% mortality rate. Others used a transfrontal or subfrontal approach to lesion the ansa lenticularis and pallidum[8-10]. Improvement in tremor and rigidity was reported in 42.5% to 70% of patients, although mortality rates were still high.

In 1952, Cooper was attempting a pedunculotomy in a young patient with post-encephalitic parkinsonism[11]. He inadvertently damaged and then ligated the anterior choroidal artery and had to abandon the planned procedure. Nonetheless, the patient experienced relief of tremor and rigidity in the contralateral limbs without motor or sensory deficits. This benefit was attributed to an ischemic lesion of the medial globus pallidus, the ansa and fasciculus lenticularis, and the ventrolateral nucleus of the thalamus[12]. Cooper went on to perform more anterior choroidal artery ligations and found this provided better relief of tremor and rigidity than earlier procedures but mortality was still 10%. Although the procedure was soon abandoned, it focused attention on the two main anatomic targets for lesioning procedures today, the thalamus and medial pallidum.

How was mortality finally reduced?

The introduction of stereotactic surgery led to a significant reduction in mortality. Stereotactic surgery entails the use of a coordinate grid system fixed in relation to the patient's head to localize an anatomic target. Spiegel and coworkers used a device consisting of a ring fixed to a plaster of Paris cap that was placed on the patient's shaved head[13]. Pneumoencephalography was used to outline the lateral ventricles which served as landmarks for target localization. Using this technique, Spiegel and Wycis lesioned the ansa lenticularis and noted reduced rigidity and tremor without weakness in four of six patients[14]. The plaster cast was later replaced by fixation pins screwed to the skull[15].

How did early thalamotomy compare to early pallidotomy?

In the 1950s both pallidotomy and thalamotomy were popular surgeries for Parkinson's disease. Thalamotomy eventually replaced pallidotomy as the procedure of choice because it reduced tremor more consistently and was associated with a lower rate of symptom recurrence. Clinical series at that time found that thalamotomy alleviated tremor in 78%-93% and rigidity in 67%-93% of cases[16-20] whereas pallidotomy alleviated tremor in 46%-82% and rigidity in 52%-90% of cases[5,19,21-23]. In addition, Cooper noted recurrence of tremor and rigidity in 25% of pallidotomy cases compared with only 11% of thalamotomy cases.

How are modern stereotactic procedures performed?

Stereotactic surgery for Parkinson's disease is typically performed using local anesthesia so that the patient can be monitored clinically and provide feedback

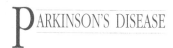

during the procedure. A stereotactic frame is initially fixed to the patient's head. An MRI or CT is then performed and target coordinates are generated. In the operating room a burr hole is placed in the skull and an electrode is advanced toward the target site. The target is then identified by electrophysiologic techniques. Macrostimulation can be used to elicit a clinical response. For thalamotomy, the target is identified as the site at which macrostimulation induces the best tremor reduction at the lowest voltage. Microelectrode recording can be used to generate more precise electrophysiologic mapping and target identification. Microelectrode recording is usually used to identify the target site for modern pallidotomy as precise targeting appears crucial. Microelectrode recording is more time consuming than stimulation alone and requires a trained electrophysiologist. Once targeting is completed a lesion is produced by application of electrothermal current.

What are the results of modern thalamotomy?

Thalamotomy is effective to reduce contralateral tremor, and to a lesser extent, rigidity. Ipsilateral tremor, bradykinesia and postural instability are not improved [24,25]. Tremor abolition has been reported in 45.8%-92% and improvement in rigidity in 41%-92% of patients [18,24-34]. Bilateral thalamotomies are reported to improve tremor in 33%-73.6% and rigidity in 22.7%-74% of patients [24,28,29,34-36]. This wide range of results is likely due to differences in surgical technique and assessment.

More recent series note short-term tremor alleviation in 90% and persistent alleviation in 82% [37]. Fox et al. used microelectrode recording to perform ventrolateral thalamotomy in 36 patients with medically refractory tremor from 1984 to 1986 [38]. They achieved persistent tremor abolition in 86% and improvement in 5%.

Are the benefits of thalamotomy permanent?

Diedrich and coworkers evaluated patients who had undergone thalamotomy a mean of 10.9 years earlier [39]. They found tremor contralateral to the thalamotomy to be significantly less than that on the opposite side, suggesting thalamotomy does produce long-term tremor suppression.

Does thalamotomy slow disease progression?

No. Disease progression continues despite thalamotomy. Over time there is a gradual worsening of rigidity, dexterity and other parkinsonian features[34].

Why do some patients lose their initial benefit?

The exact reason some patients lose benefit is not clear. Lesions that are close but not exactly on target may provide transient benefit. Functional disruption may then be followed by recovery. Whether compensatory mechanisms play a role is not known.

What are the side effects of thalamotomy?

Mortality is less than 1% and usually due to hemorrhage at the lesion site[34]. Contralateral weakness has been reported in 0.5%-26% of cases but is probably lower with the use of microelectrode recording[26,28,30-32,34,40]. Seizures occur in less than 1.3% of patients. Paresthesias, usually of the fingers or mouth, are common postoperatively but resolve within a year in all but 1%-3% of cases[24,34]. Uncommon complications include ataxia, apraxia, and gait disturbances[34].

Bilateral thalamotomy is associated with a higher incidence of speech and swallowing difficulty[41]. Tasker noted worsening of dysarthria in 29% of patients following a second thalamotomy on the opposite side[34]. Because of this, an interval of six months to a year is usually allowed before a second procedure is considered[34,35]. If speech or swallowing difficulty are still present from the first operation, a second procedure is not performed.

What is chronic thalamic stimulation?

Chronic high-frequency thalamic stimulation has recently been developed as an alternative to thalamotomy. A stimulating electrode is implanted into the ventral intermediate (VIM) nucleus of the thalamus. This is connected via a wire under the skin to a stimulator that is placed in the chest wall like a pacemaker (figure 9-1). The stimulator can be adjusted using a programmer with an electromagnetic head. The patient is able to turn the stimulator on and off using a hand-held magnet. When effective, tremor reduction occurs 1 to 3 seconds following activation of the stimulator and benefit resolves within a few seconds after deactivating the stimulator.

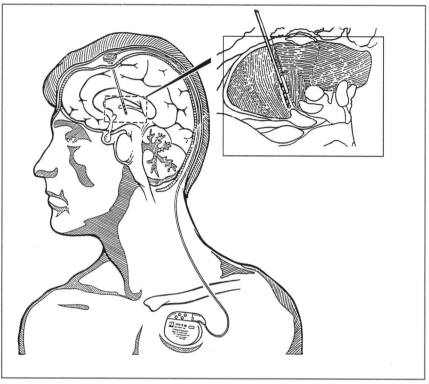

Figure 9-1. *Chronic Thalamic Stimulation. An electrode with four exposed tips is placed into the ventral intermediate (VIM) nucleus of the thalamus. The electrode is attached to a wire run beneath the skin to the stimulator placed in the chest wall.*

How was chronic thalamic stimulation developed?

Several groups were using transient high-frequency stimulation of the thalamus to identify the best site for lesioning. The site at which the least stimulation afforded the greatest tremor reduction was identified as the target. Benabid et al. proposed that chronic high-frequency stimulation might be a useful procedure for patients with disabling tremor who had previously undergone thalamotomy to avoid the potentially serious complications of bilateral thalamotomy [42]. If stimulation induced side effects it could be discontinued. Once benefit was demonstrated in this population, chronic thalamic stimulation was evaluated as an initial procedure.

What are the results of thalamic stimulation?

Chronic thalamic stimulation is effective to reduce contralateral tremor. Benabid et al. evaluated thalamic stimulation for the treatment of tremor in 26 patients[43]. Complete contralateral tremor suppression was observed in 68% and major improvement in 26%. Similarly, Blond and Siegfried reported total tremor suppression in 19 of 26 cases and improvement in the remainder[44]. Benefit has persisted through five years of follow-up. More recently, Benabid and coworkers reported results of chronic thalamic stimulation in 80 PD patients followed for up to eight years[45]. Complete or almost complete control of upper extremity tremor was achieved in 92% at three months and 88% at last follow-up. Lower extremity tremor was completely or almost completely controlled in 86% at three months and 85% at last follow-up.

What type of tremor is best controlled with thalamic stimulation?

Benabid et al. found that resting and postural tremors were better controlled than action tremors[45]. In addition, distal tremor was better controlled than proximal tremor.

What are the side effects of thalamic stimulation?

As with other stereotactic procedures, hemorrhage, stroke or death can occur, but should be limited to less than 1-2%. Most adverse effects are mild and usually resolve with discontinuation of stimulation. In the largest series to date, side effects included paresthesias (9%), dysarthria (19.6%), disequilibrium (9%), and dystonia (5%)[45]. Dysarthria was observed in 27.5% of bilaterally stimulated patients compared to 40% of those who underwent thalamotomy on one side and stimulation on the other. Of note, bilateral stimulation did not induce neuropsychological deficits usually associated with bilateral thalamotomy. These observations suggest that stimulation may be especially advantageous when bilateral procedures are contemplated.

How does thalamic stimulation work?

The mechanism of action of thalamic stimulation is not known. High-frequency stimulation may desynchronize abnormal neuronal discharges that have become overactive and autonomous[46].

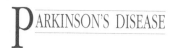
What are the relative advantages and disadvantages of thalamic stimulation?

The primary advantage of thalamic stimulation is its reversibility. If stimulation produces a side effect the stimulation parameters can be adjusted, or if necessary, stimulation can be discontinued. The primary disadvantages are the increased cost and possible need to replace the battery. The battery life of current stimulators is several years but this may be improved in the future. Another potential disadvantage is the possibility of infection or fracture of the implanted system. How often this might occur is not yet known.

Which patients are candidates for chronic thalamic stimulation?

Patients with functional disability due to medically refractory tremor are candidates for chronic thalamic stimulation. This procedure does not improve other parkinsonian features such as rigidity or incoordination. Patients will only experience functional improvement with regard to disability caused by tremor alone.

What is pallidotomy?

Pallidotomy is the lesioning of the globus pallidus interna (GPi).

What rekindled interest in pallidotomy?

Thalamotomy overshadowed pallidotomy in the 1950s because it relieved tremor more consistently (90% vs. 60%). In the 1980s, increased understanding of the functional anatomy of the basal ganglia motor circuit rekindled interest in pallidotomy and forced a re-evaluation of prior work.

What does the basal ganglia motor circuit tell us about target sites for surgery for Parkinson's disease?

The striatum receives input from the cortex. Striatal output is directed to the medial globus pallidus (GPi) through two pathways, a direct striatopallidal pathway and an indirect pathway through the external segment of the globus pallidus (GPe) and the subthalamic nucleus (figure 1-3). Output from the GPi exerts an inhibitory effect on thalamocortical neurons and decreases output from the motor cortex. In Parkinson's disease, loss of substantia nigra neurons leads to decreased dopamine levels in the striatum. Decreased striatal dopamine diminishes inhibition of the GPi via the direct pathway and increases stimulation of the GPi via the indirect pathway (figure 1-4). The result is increased firing by the GPi and increased inhibition of the thalamocortical pathway. Thus, decreased striatal dopamine causes increased inhibition of the thalamocortical pathway by the GPi and results in decreased output from the motor cortex. This may cause bradykinesia and rigidity in Parkinson's disease.

Inspection of the basal ganglia circuitry suggests two rational targets for lesioning surgery. The outflow of the basal ganglia circuitry is through the medial globus pallidus (GPi). In Parkinson's disease, the GPi is overfiring, resulting in thalamocortical inhibition. A lesion of the GPi would abolish overfiring of the GPi and eliminate the increased inhibition of the thalamocortical pathway (figure 9-2). This might improve bradykinesia and rigidity. Another possible target for lesioning is the subthalamic nucleus, part of the indirect pathway. The subthalamic nucleus (STN) is also overfiring in Parkinson's disease and an STN lesion would reduce stimulation of the GPi via the indirect pathway (figure 9-3).

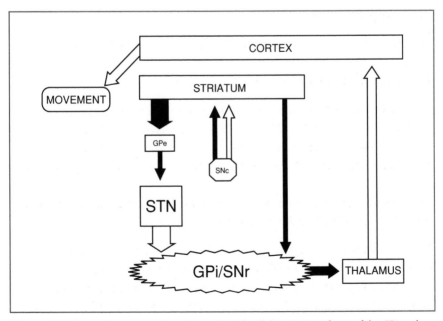

Figure 9-2. *Schematic representation of the effect of pallidotomy. Overfiring of the GPi and resultant excessive inhibition of the thalamocortical patyhway are returned toward normal. See text for details.*

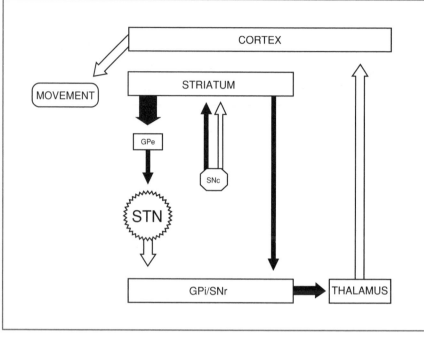

Figure 9-3. *Schematic representation of the effect of subthalamic nucleus lesioning. STN-driven overfiring of the GPi and resultant excessive inhibition of the thalamocortical pathway are returned toward normal.*

How was pallidotomy "rediscovered"?

In the 1950s, Leksell found pallidotomy using the usual target in the anterodorsal pallidum to be unsatisfactory and he moved his target to the posteroventral pallidum. Evaluation of 81 cases through 1957 suggested long-term tremor suppression in 82% and relief of rigidity in 79% [22]. Of the last 20 patients to undergo posteroventral pallidotomy, 19 were reported to experience persistent relief of tremor and rigidity. Improvement in bradykinesia was also noted. Although Leksell continued to perform pallidotomies from 1958 to 1962 he never published this series.

Based on discussions with Leksell, Laitinen began performing posteroventral pallidotomy in 1985. In 38 patients whose main complaint was hypokinesia, long-term tremor relief was reported in 81% and complete or almost complete relief of rigidity and hypokinesia was reported in 92% [47,48]. Speech, gait, dystonia, and levodopa-induced dyskinesias were also improved.

What are the results of modern pallidotomy?

Dogali et al. reported results of stereotactic ventral pallidotomy using microelectrode recording in 18 patients with severe motor fluctuations [49]. Following lesioning, improvement was noted in bradykinesia, rigidity, resting tremor, and balance with resolution of contralateral levodopa-induced dyskinesia. Patients were able to tolerate larger levodopa doses due to reduced dyskinesia. The greatest improvements were seen while patients were "off". At twelve months, parkinson scores (UPDRS) while off were improved by 65%, and timed tests of motor function were improved 38.2% in the contralateral limb and 24.2% in the ipsilateral limb. Walking scores improved 45%. Improvements were also noted during "best on" although these were much less striking than those during off periods. Similar benefit has been reported by others [50].

Baron et al. [51] recently reported results of posterior GPi pallidotomy in fifteen patients with advanced PD. Significant improvement was observed in ADL and motor scores during the "off" state one year following surgery. ADL "off" scores were improved at three months (34.1%, p= .008) and one year (14.9%, p= 0.035). Motor "off" scores were also improved at three months (24.9%, p= 0.001) and one year (21.3%, p= 0.002). All cardinal features were improved and contralateral drug-induced dyskinesias were dramatically ameliorated. ADL and motor scores during the "on" state were only transiently improved.

How long does it take for pallidotomy to have an effect?

The effect of pallidotomy is immediate and often observed during the operation.

What are the side effects of pallidotomy?

Because the optic tract and internal capsule lie in close proximity to the GPi, potential complications include visual field deficits and hemiparesis. The use of microelectrode recording has greatly diminished the incidence of these side effects. Although catastrophic events can and do still occur, most complications of modern pallidotomy are mild and transient. These include dysphagia, dysarthria, facial droop, worsened handwriting, visual field defects, weight gain, confusion, and somnolence [49,51].

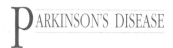

Which patients are the best candidates for pallidotomy?

Ideal candidates for pallidotomy are relatively young, cognitively intact, and maintaining a good response to levodopa although with severe motor fluctuations and dyskinesia. Dyskinesia is the symptom most consistently and dramatically improved by pallidotomy. Baron et al. found that patient age inversely correlated with improvement in total UPDRS scores at three months. Scores decreased by an average of 52.2% in younger patients (38-52 years) and by 13.8% in older patients (58-69 years) [51].

How would you summarize the results of pallidotomy to date?

There is only limited information available on the short-term effects of modern pallidotomy and almost none on its long-term effects. Nonetheless, it seems clear that in the right hands, pallidotomy is very effective to alleviate contralateral dyskinesia. In addition, pallidotomy may afford improvement in the signs of Parkinson's disease, especially in the contralateral limbs during off periods. However, Baron et al. noted only 21% improvement in motor "off" scores at one year in their open label study [51]. Function in the "on" state (other than dyskinesia) does not appear improved.

Can chronic stimulation be applied to the pallidum?

Yes. Very preliminary results suggest that bilateral chronic stimulation of the pallidum may be a viable alternative to pallidal lesioning [52].

Is the subthalamic nucleus a target for stereotactic surgery?

Knowledge of the functional anatomy of the basal ganglia suggests that the subthalamic nucleus is a rational target for surgery in Parkinson's disease. Very preliminary experience offers hope that lesioning or stimulation of the subthalamic nucleus may provide beneficial effects [53].

What is the concept behind transplantation as a surgical treatment for Parkinson's disease?

The basic idea of transplantation is to replace lost dopaminergic neurons.

Why is Parkinson's disease an attractive target for transplantation?

Parkinson's disease is an attractive target disease for transplantation because the degeneration is relatively site and neuron specific (dopaminergic neurons of the nigrostriatal pathway), the striatal implantation area is relatively large, and clinical benefit can be attained with neurotransmitter replacement rather than being dependent on restoration of neuronal circuitry.

Do animal studies indicate that transplantation is a viable procedure?

Studies in animal models of Parkinson's disease have demonstrated that transplanted fetal mesencephalic neurons survive, form synaptic connections, exhibit normal firing patterns, and improve parkinsonian features [54-65]. These studies also indicate that implantation of appropriate tissue into an appropriate location is necessary for clinical benefit.

What was the first transplantation strategy employed in Parkinson's disease?

Autologous adrenal medullary transplantation was the first transplant strategy used in Parkinson's disease because it was not encumbered by the logistic, ethical and immunologic issues surrounding fetal cell transplantation. In animal studies, adrenal cell transplantation was found to provide some benefit although this was limited and not as great as was observed using fetal tissue.

What were the results of adrenal transplantation in Parkinson's disease patients?

The first attempts at adrenal transplantation began in 1982 and were found to bring about only minimal and transient improvement [66,67]. However, in 1987, Madrazo and coworkers reported "dramatic amelioration" of symptoms in two young patients [68]. Subsequent investigators noted only modest improvement in function during off time and a mild reduction of off time [69-78]. Most of this benefit was lost by two years [79]. Patients who came to autopsy were found to have few or no surviving transplanted cells [73,80-83]. This procedure has now been abandoned.

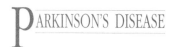

If transplanted adrenal cells do not survive, what is the mechanism of benefit?

The possibility of a placebo effect cannot be totally eliminated. However, as was seen in animal studies, there was evidence of increased dopaminergic function in host tissue near the site of implantation [83,84]. This could possibly be due to trophic factors associated with the graft or the trauma from surgery itself.

What are the important technical issues concerning fetal transplantation?

There are many unanswered questions concerning issues in fetal transplantation that might influence clinical outcome. These include source of tissue, donor tissue age, amount of tissue grafted, tissue preparation and storage, need for immunosuppression, and when in the course of the disease to transplant.

Two of the most critical issues are donor age and amount of tissue transplanted. The optimal donor age appears to be between 6 and 8 weeks post-ovulation [85,86]. Cell survival is generally not seen with tissue older than 10 to 12 weeks. In addition, there has been a trend to transplant greater amounts of tissue in an effort to maximize clinical benefit.

What were the results of the first attempts at fetal grafting in Parkinson's disease?

Lindvall and coworkers first evaluated fetal grafting in two patients using a mesencephalic cell suspension from single donors [87,88]. These patients experienced modest but significant improvement in motor function while off. Two additional patients received cell suspension grafts from four donors [89,90]. These patients experienced gradual improvement beginning 6 to 12 weeks after surgery. Motor function while off progressively improved and off time decreased. Improvement in bradykinesia and rigidity was observed bilaterally but was most pronounced on the contralateral side. Fluorodopa PET studies demonstrated improved dopaminergic function beginning one year after transplant [91]. This experience indicated that clinical improvement may be dependent on transplanting a sufficient amount of tissue. Several other groups have also reported modest benefit with transplant using a single donor [92-94].

In contrast, more benefit was observed in two patients with MPTP-induced parkinsonism [95]. These patients received bilateral transplants using tissue from 3-4 donors per side. It is possible that greater improvement occurred because these patients had MPTP-induced parkinsonism rather than Parkinson's disease. Alternatively, they may have experienced more benefit due to the greater amount of tissue transplanted.

What are the results of recent fetal cell transplantation?

Freeman and coworkers recently reported their experience with fetal transplantation in four patients [96]. Solid grafts were implanted bilaterally using 3-4 donors per side. All patients experienced clinically meaningful benefit. Significant improvement was noted in parkinson (UPDRS) and disability scores while off. Both off time and on time with dyskinesia were significantly reduced. Fluorodopa uptake by PET scan improved by a mean of 43%.

One patient died 18 months after surgery due to an unrelated cause [97]. He had experienced sustained improvement in motor function and a progressive increase in fluorodopa uptake on PET scan. On examination of the brain, each of the large grafts was viable, contained dense clusters of dopaminergic neurons, and was well integrated into the host striatum. Processes from these neurons had grown out from the grafts to reinnervate the striatum. This case demonstrates that grafted mesencephalic tissue can survive for a long period and restore dopaminergic innervation.

What is the future of fetal transplantation for Parkinson's disease?

Several large prospective randomized controlled studies of fetal transplantation for Parkinson's disease are now underway. These studies should more clearly define the benefits of transplantation as it currently exists. At the same time there will be attempts to improve the technique of transplantation. We anticipate the use of greater amounts of donor tissue and moving the procedure earlier into the disease. It is hoped that transplantation earlier in the disease may delay or prevent the development of fluctuations and dyskinesia.

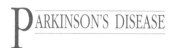

What is the future of transplantation?

The ideal tissue source should be readily available, non-immunogenic, and inexpensive. Attempts at cross-species grafting are underway. An alternative approach is the development of genetically modified cell lines for transplantation. Cell lines can potentially be modified to increase dopamine production or release of trophic factors. In fact, it might be possible to use viral vectors to directly modify host cells to increase dopamine production or limit further degeneration.

How would you summarize the results of fetal transplantation?

Moderate benefit has been observed. Function during off periods is improved, off time is reduced, and dyskinesia is reduced. Whether greater benefit can be achieved with improvements in transplantation technique is uncertain.

How do the results of fetal transplant compare with pallidotomy?

The effects of pallidotomy are evident immediately whereas the benefits of transplantation are seen after several months. Transplant's greatest benefit may be a reduction of off time whereas pallidotomy may have little effect on the amount of off time. Both procedures are reported to improve function during off periods.

How would you summarize current procedures for Parkinson's disease?

Surgeries for Parkinson's disease should be performed only at centers with expert teams of clinicians. Except in clinical studies, surgery should be reserved for patients who are disabled by medically refractory symptoms.

Thalamotomy is an appropriate procedure for patients with medically intractable tremor. It has little effect on symptoms other than tremor. Chronic thalamic stimulation appears to be an effective alternative to thalamotomy. As stimulation is adjustable, it may afford improved safety, especially for patients who may need bilateral procedures.

Pallidotomy appears to be very effective in alleviating contralateral dyskinesia and effective in improving parkinsonian features, especially in contralateral limbs during off periods. The best candidates are those who are young, cognitively intact, and maintaining a good response to levodopa although with severe fluctuations and/or dyskinesia.

Fetal transplant improves function during off periods and reduces off time. Ideal candidates are similar to those for pallidotomy. Advances in the transplant procedure offer hope that more benefit can be achieved in the future.

What should I tell patients who are considering surgery?

Patients need to be informed that surgery carries real risk of morbidity and mortality. In general, stereotactic surgery is associated with major morbidity and mortality of up to one percent. In addition, there is no guarantee of benefit. Every effort should be made to reduce disability by non-surgical means before surgery is contemplated.

For the timebeing, patients need to expect that they will only be able to undergo one type of procedure during their lifetime. They should carefully consider when surgery is an appropriate option and which procedure best matches their symptoms. In addition, the experience of the surgeon and the rest of the clinical team are vitally important.

PARKINSON'S DISEASE

REFERENCES

Chapter 1 references

1. Parkinson J. An essay on the shaking palsy. London; Sherwood, Neely & Jones 1817, 66.

2. Duvoisin RC. History of parkinsonism. Pharmacology and Therapeutics 1987;32:1-17.

3. Martilla RJ, Rinne UK. Epidemiological approaches to the etiology of Parkinson's disease. Acta Neurol Scand 1989;126:13-18.

4. Martilla RJ, Rinne UK. Epidemiology of Parkinson's disease in Finland. Acta Neurol Scand 1976;53(2);81-102.

5. Lilienfeld DE, Chan E, Ehland J, Godbold J, Landrigan PH, Marsh G, Perl DP. Two decades of increasing mortality from Parkinson's disease among the US elderly. Arch Neurol 1990;47:731-734.

6. Rajput AH, Offord K, Beard CM, Kurland LT. Epidemiology of Parkinsonism: incidence, classification, and mortality. Ann Neurol 1984;16:278-282.

7. Bharucha NE, Bharucha EP, Bharucha AE, Bhise AV, Schoenberg BS. Prevalence of Parkinson's disease in the Parsi community of Bombay, India. Arch Neurol 1988;45:1321-1323.

8. Kessler II. Epidemiologic studies of Parkinson's disease. American J of Epi 1972;95:308-318.

9. Cosnett JE, Bill PL. Parkinson's disease in blacks. Observations on epidemiology in Natal. South African Medical Journal 1988;73:281-3.

10. Schoenberg BS, Anderson DW, Haerer AF. Prevalence of Parkinson's disease in the biracial population of Copiah County, Mississippi. Neurology 1985;35:841-845.

11. Manyam BV. Paralysis agitans and levodopa in "Ayurveda": ancient Indian medical treatise. Movement Disorders 1990;5:47-8.

12. Ballard PA, Tetrud JW, Langston JW. Permanent human parkinsonism due to 1-methyl-4-phenyl-1,2,3,6-tetrahydropyridine (MPTP): seven cases. Neurology 1985;35:949-956.

13. Hoehn MM. The natural history of Parkinson's disease in the pre-levodopa and post-levodopa eras. In: Cedarbaum JM, Gancher ST eds. Neurologic Clinics. Philadelphia PA: W.B. Saunders and Company 1992;331.

14. Wichman T, DeLong M. Pathophysiology of parkinsonian motor abnormalities. In: Narabayashi H, Nagatsu T, Yanagisawa N, Mizuno Y. Advances in Neurology New York: Raven Press 1993;53-60.

15. Gibb WRG. Neuropathology of movement disorders. J Neurol Neurosurg Psych 1989;55-67.

16. Nagatsu T. Biochemical aspects of Parkinson's disease. In: Narabayashi H, Nagatsu T, Yanagisawa N, Mizuno Y. Advances in Neurology New York: Raven Press 1993;165-174.

17. Agid Y, Cervera P, Hirsch E, Javoy-Agid F, Lehericy S, Raisman R, Ruberg M. Biochemistry of Parkinson's disease 28 years later: a critical review. Movement Disorders 1989;4:S126-44.

18. Goldstein M, Lieberman A. The role of the regulatory enzymes of catecholamine synthesis in Parkinson's disease. Neurology 1992;42:8-12

19. Sibley DR, Monsma FJ Jr. Molecular biology of dopamine receptors. Trends Pharmacol Sci 1992;13:61-9.

20. Kebabian JW, Calne DB. Multiple receptors for dopamine. Nature 1979;277:93-96.

21. Calne DB. Treatment of Parkinson's disease. New Eng J Med 1993;3239:1021-1027.

22. Brooks DJ, Ibanez V, Sawle GV, et al. Differing patterns of striatal 18F-dopa uptake in Parkinson's disease, multiple system atrophy, and progressive supranuclear palsy. Ann Neurol 1990;28:547-55.

23. Brucke T, Kornhuber J, Angelberger P, Asenbaum S, Frassine H, Podreka I. SPECT imaging of dopamine and serotonin transporters with [123I] beta-CIT. Binding kinetics in the human brain. J Neurol Transm 1993;94:137-46.

Chapter 2 references

1. Calne DB, Stoessl AJ. Early parkinsonism. Clinical Neuropharmacology 1986;9:S3-8.

2. Calne DB, Snow BJ, Lee C. Criteria for diagnosing Parkinson's disease. Ann Neurol 1992;32:S125-127.

3. Gibb WRG, Lees AJ. The clinical phenomenon of akathisia. J Neur Neurosurg Psych 1986;49:861-866.

4. Hoehn MM, Yahr MD. Parkinsonism: onset, progression and mortality. Neurology 1967;17:427-442.

5. Gibb WRG, Lees AJ. A comparison of clinical and pathological features of young- and old-onset Parkinson's disease. Neurology 1988;38:1402-1406.

6. Diagnostic and Statistical Manual of Mental Disorders, fourth edition. American Psychiatric Association Washington D.C. 1994;134.

7. Brown RG, Marsden CD. How common is dementia in Parkinson's disease? The Lancet 1984;56;1262-1265.

8. Lieberman A, Dziatolowski M, Kupersmith M, Serby M, Goodgold A, Korein J, and Goldstein M. Dementia in Parkinson's disease. Ann Neurol 1979;6:355-359.

9. Cummings JL. The dementias of Parkinson's disease: prevalence, characteristics, neurobiology, and comparison with dementia of the Alzheimer type. Eur Neurol 1988;28:15-23.

10. Agid Y, Ruberg M, Dubois B et al. Parkinson's disease and dementia. Clin Neuropharm 1986;9:S22-36.

11. Cummings JL. Depression and Parkinson's disease: a review. Am J Psychiatry 1992;149:443-454.

12. Mayeux R, Stern Y, Williams JBW, Cote L, Frantz A, Dyrenfurth I. Clinical and biochemical features of depression in Parkinson's disease. Am J Psychiatry 1986;143:756-759.

13. Awerbuch GI. Autonomic functions in the early stages of Parkinson's disease. Intern J Neuroscience 1992;64:7-14.

14. Turkka JT, Tolonen U, Myllyla VV. Cardiovascular reflexes in Parkinson's disease. European Neurology 1987;26:104-12.

15. Langston JW, Forno LS. The hypothalamus in Parkinson's disease. Ann Neurol 1978;3:129-133.

16. Laihinen A, Alihanka J, Raitasuo S, Rinne UK. Sleep movements and associated autonomic nervous activities in patients with Parkinson's disease. Acta Neurol Scand 1987;76:64-68.

17. Mouret J. Differences in sleep in patients with Parkinson's disease. Electroencephalography & Clinical Neurophysiology. 1975;38:653-7.

18. Fahn S, Elton RL, Members of the UPDRS Development Committee. Unified Parkinson's disease rating scale. In: Fahn S, Marsden CD, Calne DB, Goldstein M, Eds. Recent developments in Parkinson's disease. Vol 2. Florham Park, NJ: Macmillan Health Care Information 1987, 153-164.

Chapter 3 references

1. Schou M, Baastrup PC, Grof P, Weis P, Angst J. Pharmacological and clinical problems of lithium prophylaxis. Br J Psych 1970;116:615-619.

2. Yamadori A, Albert M. Involuntary movement disorder caused by methyldopa. N Eng J Med 1972;286:610.

3. Rajput AH, Rozdilsky B, Hornykiewicz O et al. Reversible drug-induced parkinsonism. Arch Neurol 1982;39:644-646.

4. Logan WJ, Freeman JM. Pseudodegenerative disease due to diphenylhydantoin intoxication. Arch Neurol 1969;21:631-637.

5. Karas BJ, Wilder BJ, Hammond EJ et al. Treatment of valproate tremors. Neurology 1983;33:1380-1382.

6. Gibb WRG. Accuracy in the clinical diagnosis of parkinsonian syndromes. Postgraduate Med Jour 1988;64:345-351.

7. Ballard PA, Tetrud JW, Langston JW. Permanent human parkinsonism due to 1-methyl-4-phenyl-1,2,3,6-tetrahydropyridine (MPTP): seven cases. Neurology 1985;35:949-956.

8. Tolosa ES, Santamaria J. Parkinsonism and basal ganglia infarcts. Neurology 1984;34:1516-8.

9. Ferbert A, Gerwig M. Tremor due to stroke. Movement Disorders 1993;8:179-182.

10. Duvoisin RC, Yahr MD. Encephalitis and parkinsonism. Arch Neurol 1965;12:227-239.

11. Ziegler LH. Follow-up studies on persons who have had epidemic encephalitis. JAMA 1928;91:138-141.

12. Martland JS. Punch drunk. JAMA 1928;91:1103-7.

13. Corselis JAN, Bruton CJ, Freeman-Browne D. The aftermath of boxing. Psychol Med 1973;3:270-303.

14. Larsen TA, Calne DB. Essential tremor. Clin Neuropharmacol 1983;6:185-206.

15. Critchley M. Observations on essential (heredofamilial) tremor. Brain 1949;72:113-39.

16. Larson T, Sjogren T. Essential tremor. A clinical and genetic population study. Acta Psychiatr Neurol Scand 1960;36:1-176.

17. Koller WC, Busenbark K, Gray C, Hassanein RS, Dubinsky R. Classification of essential tremor. Clin Neurophar 1992;15:81-87.

18. Wilson SAK. Progressive lenticular degeneration: a familial nervous disease associated with cirrhosis of the liver. Brain 1912;34:295-507.

19. Levine IM, Estes JW, Looney JM. Hereditary neurological disease with acanthocytosis. A new syndrome. Arch Neurol 1968;19:403-409.

20. Aminoff MJ. Acanthocytosis and neurological disease. Brain 1972;95:749-760.

21. Sotaniemi KA. Chorea acanthocythosis-neurologic disease with acanthocytosis. Acta Neurol Scand 1983;68:53-56.

22. Huntington G. On Chorea. Lea and Blanchard, Philadelphia, Medical and Surgical Reporter 1872;26:317.

23. Hayden MR. Huntington's chorea. New York, Springer-Verlag, 1981.

24. Huntington's Disease Collaborative Research Group. A novel gene containing a trinucleotide repeat that is expanded and unstable on Huntington's disease chromosomes. Cell 1993;72:971-983.

25. Klawans HL, Weiner WJ. The pharmacology of choreatic movement disorder. Prog Neurobiol 1976;6:49-80.

26. Steele JC, Richardson JC, Olszewski J. Progressive supranuclear palsy. Arch Neurol 1964;10:333-359.

27. Golbe LI, Davis PH, Schoenberg BS, Duvoisin RC. Prevalence and natural history of progressive supranuclear palsy. Neurology 1988;38:1031-1034.

28. Jankovic J, Friedman DI, Pirozzolo FJ, McCrary JA. Progressive supranuclear palsy: motor, neurobahavioral, and neuro-ophthalmic findings. In: Streifler MB, Korczyn AD, Melamed E, Youdim MBH, Advances in Neurology; Raven Press, New York, 1990.

29. Fukushima-Kudo J, Fukushima K, Tashiro K. Rigidity and dorsiflexion of the neck in progressive supranuclear palsy and the interstitial nucleus of Cajal. J Neurol Neurosurg Psychiatry 1987;50:1197-1203.

30. Pillon B, Dubois B, Lhermitte F, Agid Y. Heterogeneity of cognitive impairment in progressive supranuclear palsy, Parkinson's disease, and Alzheimer's disease. Neurology 1986;36:1179-1185.

31. Oppenheimer DR. Diseases of the basal ganglia, cerebellum and motorneurons. In Blackwood W, Corsellis JAN Eds: Greenfield's Neuropathology. London, Edward Arnold 1976:608-651.

32. Quinn N. Multiple system atrophy-the nature of the beast. J Neurol Neurosurg Psychiatry 1989;52:78-79.

33. Shy GM, Drager GA. A neurological syndrome associated with orthostatic hypotension: a clinical-pathological study. Arch Neurol 1960;2:511-527.

34. Rajput AH, Rozdilsky B. Dysautonomia in parkinsonism: a clinicopathological study. J Neurol Neurosurg Psychiatry 1976;39:1092-1100.

35. Lees AJ, Bannister R. The use of lisuride in the treatment of multiple system atrophy with autonomic failure (Shy-Drager syndrome). J Neurol Neurosurg Psychiatry 1981;44:347-351.

36. Dejerine J, Thomas A. L'atrophie olivo-ponto-cerebelleuses. Nouv Iconogr Salpet 1900;13:330-370.

37. Berciano J. Olivopontocerebellar atrophy. J Neurol Sci 1982;53:253-272.

38. Lees AJ, Bannister R. The use of lisuride in the treatment of multiple system atrophy with autonomic failure (Shy-Drager syndrome). J Neurol Neurosurg Psychiatry 1982;44:347-351.

39. Koeppen AH, Barron KD. The neuropathology of olivopontocerebellar atrophy. In: Duvoisin RC, Plaitakis A Eds: The Olivopontocerebellar Atrophies. New York, Raven Press 1984:13-38.

40. Huang YP, Plaitakis A. Morphological changes of olivopontocerebellar atrophy in computed tomography and comments on its pathogenesis. In Duvoisin RC, Plaitakis A Eds: The Olivopontocerebellar Atrophies. New York, Raven Press 1984:39-85.

41. Adams RD, Van Bogaert L, Van Der Eecken H. Striatonigral degeneration. J Neuropath Exp Neruol 1964;23:584-608.

42. Takei Y, Samuels NS. Striatonigral degeneration: a form of multiple system atrophy with clinical parkinsonism. In: Zimmerman HM Ed: Progress in Neuropathology Vol 2. New York, Grune and Stratton 1973, 217-251.

43. Reibeiz JJ, Kolodny EH, Richardson E. Corticodentatonigral degeneration with neuronal achromasia. Arch Neurol 1968;18:20-33.

44. Riley DE, Lang AE, Lewis A, et al. Cortical-basal ganglionic degeneration. Neurology 1990;40:1203-1212.

45. Case records of the Massachusetts General Hospital. N Engl J Med 1985;313:739-748.

46. Louis ED, Goldman JE, Powers JM, Fahn S. Parkinsonian features of eight pathologically diagnosed cases of diffuse Lewy body disease. Movement Disorders 1994;10:188-94.

47. Hansen LA, Galasko D. Lewy body disease. Current Opinion in Neurology & Neurosurgery. 1992;5:889-94.

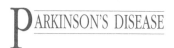

Chapter 4 references

1. Carlsson A, Winblad B. Influence of age and time interval between death and autopsy on dopamine and 3-methoxytyramine levels in human basal ganglia. J Neural Transm 1976; 38:271-276.

2. Purjol J, Junque C, Vendrell P, Grau JM, Capdevila A. Reduction of the substantia nigra width and motor decline in aging and Parkinson's disease. Arch Neurol 1992;49:1119-1122.

3. Calne DB, Peppard RF. Aging of the nigrostriatal pathway in humans. Can J Neurol Sci 1987;14:424-427.

4 . Fearnley JM, Lees AJ. Aging and Parkinson's disease: substantia nigra regional selectivity. Brain 1991;114:2283-301.

5. Koller W, O'Hara R, Weiner W, et al. Relationship of aging to Parkinson's disease. Adv Neurol 1986;45:317-321.

6. Neuman RP, LeWitt PA, Jaffe M, Calne DB, Larsen TA. Motor function in the normal aging population; treatment with levodopa. Neurology 1985;35:571-573.

7. Agid Y, Cervera P, Hirsch E, Javoy-Agid F, Lehericy S, Raisman R, Ruberg M. Biochemistry of Parkinson's disease 28 years later: a critical review. Movement Disorders 1989:4;S126-144.

8. Sawle GV, Colebatch JG, Shah A, Brooks DJ, Marsden CD, Frackowiak RSJ. Striatal function in normal aging: implications for Parkinson's disease. Ann Neurol 1990;28:799-804.

9. Duvoisin RC. Genetics of Parkinson's disease. In: Yahr MD, Bergmann KJ eds. Adv Neurol 45, Parkinson's Disease. New York, Raven Press, 1987, 307-312.

10. Ward CD, Duvoisin RC, Ince SE, et al. Parkinson's disease in 65 pairs of twins and in a set of quadruplets. Neurology 1983:33:815-824.

11. Burn DJ, Mark MH, Playford ED, et al. Parkinson's disease in twins studied with F-dopa and positron emission tomography. Neurology 1992;42:1894-1900.

12. Polymeropoulos MH, Higgins JJ, Golbe LI, et al. Mapping of a gene for Parkinson's disease to chromosome 4q21-q23. Science 1996;274:1197-1199.

13. Globe LI, Di Iorio G, Samges G, et al. Clinical genetic analysis of Parkinson's disease in the Contursi kindred. Annals of Neurology 1996;40:767-775.

14. Schwartz J, Elizan T. Search for viral particles and virus-specific products in idiopathic Parkinson's disease brain material. Ann Neurol 1979;6:261-263.

15. Martilla RJ, Rinne UK, Halonen P, Madden DL, Sever JL. Herpes viruses and parkinsonism. Arch Neurol 1981;38:19-21.

16. Sasco AJ, Paffenbarger RS. Measles infection and Parkinson's disease. Am J Epidemiol 1985;122:1017-31.

17. Mattock C, Marmot M, Stern G. Could Parkinson's disease follow intra-uterine influenza - a speculative hypothesis. J Neurol Neurosurg Psychiatry 1988;51:753-756.

18. Earle KM. Studies on Parkinson's disease including x-ray fluorescence spectroscopy of formalin fixed brain tissue. J Neuropath Exp Neurol 1968;27:1-14.

19. Sian J, Dexter DT, Lees AJ, et al. Alterations in glutathione levels in Parkinson's disease and other neurodegenerative disorders affecting basal ganglia. Ann Neurol 1994;36:348-355.

20. Gerlach M, Ben-Shachar D, Riederer P, Youdim MBH. Altered brain metabolism of iron as a cause of neurodegenerative diseases? J Neurochem 1994;63(3):793-807.

21. Youdim MB, Ben-Shachar D, Riederer P. The enigma of neuromelanin in Parkinson's disease substantia nigra. J Neurol Trans 1994;43:113-22.

22. Kalra J, Rajput AH, Mantha SV, Chaudhary AK, Prasad K. Oxygen free radical producing activity of polymorphonuclear leukocytes in patients with Parkinson's disease. Molecular and Cellular Biochemistry 1992;112:181-6.

23. Przedborski S, Kostic V, Jackson-Lewis V, et al. Transgenic mice with increased Cu/Zn-superoxide dismutase activity are resistant to N-methyl-4-phenyl-1,2,3,6-tetrahydropyridine-induced neurotoxicity. J Neurosci 1992;12:1658-1667.

24. Hirsch EC. Why are nigral catecholaminergic neurons more vulnerable than other cells in Parkinson's disease? Ann Neurol 1992;32:S88-93.

25. Zhang P, Damier P, Hirsch EC, et al. Preferential expression of superoxide dismutase messenger RNA in melanized neurons in human mesencephalon. Neurosci 1993;55:167-175.

26. Checkoway H, Costa LG, Woods JS, Castoldi AF, Lund BO, Swanson PD. Peripheral blood cell activities of monoamine oxidase B and superoxide dismutase in Parkinson's disease. J Neurol Trans 1992;4:283-90.

27. Davis GC, Williams AC, Markey SP, Ebert MH, Caine ED, Reichert CM, Kopin IJ. Chronic parkinsonism secondary to intravenous injection of meperidine analogues. Psychiatry Research 1979;1:249-254.

28. Ballard PA, Tetrud JW, Langston JW. Permanent human parkinsonism due to 1-methyl-4-phenyl-1,2,3,6-tetrahydropyridine (MPTP): seven cases. Neurology 1985;35:949-956.

29. Davey GP, Tipton KF, Murphy MP. Uptake and accumulation of 1-methyl-4-phenylpyridinium by rat liver mitochondria measured using an ion-selective electrode. Biochem Med J 1992;288:439-43.

30. Schapira AH, Mann VM, Cooper JM, et al. Anatomic and disease specificity of NADH CoQ1 reductase (complex 1) deficiency in Parkinson's disease. J Neurochem 1990;55:2142-2145.

31. Haas RH, Nsairian F, Nakano K, Ward D, Pay M, Hill R, Shults CW. Low platelet mitochondrial complex I and complex II/III activity in early untreated Parkinson's disease. Ann Neurol 1995;37:714-22.

32. Benecke R, Strumper P, Weiss H. Electron transfer complexes I and IV of platelets are abnormal in Parkinson's disease but normal in Parkinson-plus syndromes. Brain 1993;116:1451-1463.

33. Kessler II. Epidemiologic studies of Parkinson's disease. 3. A community-based survey. American Journal of Epidemiology 1972;96:242-54.

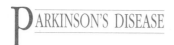
34. Shults CW. Future Perfect? Presymptomatic diagnosis, neural transplantation, and trophic factors. In: Cedarbaum JM, Gancher ST eds. Neurologic Clinics Philadelphia, PA:WB Saunders 1992;567-593.

35. Lin LF, Doherty DH, Lile JD, Bektesh S, Collins F. GDNF: a glial cell line-derived neurotrophic factor for midbrain dopaminergic neurons. Science 1993;260:1130-1132.

36. Lindsay R, Thoenen H, Barde YA. Placode and neural crest-derived sensory neurons are responsible at early developmental stages to brain-derived neurotrophic factors. Developmental Biology 1985;112:319-28.

37. Hynes MA, Poulson K, Armanini M, Berkemeier L, Phillips H, Rosenthal A. Neurotrophin-4/5 is a survival factor for embryonic midbrain dopaminergic neurons in enriched cultures. J Neurosci Res 1994;37:144-154.

Chapter 5 references

1. Cotzias GC, Van Woert MH, Shiffer LM. Aromatic amino acids and modification of parkinsonism. N Engl J Med 1967;276:347-379.

2. Carlsson A. The occurrence, distribution, and physiological role of catecholamines in the nervous system. Pharmacol Rev 1959;11:490-493.

3. Ehringer, H, Hornykiewicz O. Vertelung von noradrenalin und dopamin (3-hydroxytyramin) im gehirn des menschen und ihr verhalten bei erkrankum gen des extrapyramidalen systems. Klin Wschr 1960;38:1236-1239.

4. Cotzias GC, Papavasilou PS, Gellene R. Experimental treatment of parkinsonism with L-dopa. Neurology 1968;18:276-7.

5. Bartholini GJ, Pletscher A. Effects of various decarboxylase inhibitors on the cerebral metabolism of dihydroxyphenylalanine. J Pharamacol 1969;21:323-324.

6. Kurlan R, Rothfield AB, Woodward WR, Nutt JG, Miller C, Lichter D, and Shoulson I. Erratic gastric empting of levodopa may cause "random" fluctuations of parkinsonian mobility. Neurology 1988;48:419-421.

7. Leon AS, Spiegel HE. The effect of antacid administration on the absorption and metabolism of levodopa. J Clinical Pharmacol 1972;12:263-267.

8. Nutt JG, Fellman JH. Pharmacokinetics of levodopa. Clin Neuropharm 1984;7:35-49.

9. Physicians Desk Reference 50th ed, 1996. Medical Economics Company, Montvale, NJ.

10. Pittner H, Stormann H, Enzenhofer R. Pharmacodynamic actions of midodrine, a new a-adrenergic stimulating agent, and its main metabolite, ST 1059. Arzneim Forsch 1976;26:2145-2154.

11. Goetz CG, Tanner CM, Klawans HL et al. Parkinson's disease and motor fluctuations: long-acting carbidopa/levodopa (CR4-Sinemet). Neurology 1987;37:875-878.

12. Yeh KC, August TF, Bush DF et al. Pharmacokinetics and bioavailability of Sinemet CR: a summary of human studies. Neurology 1989;39:S25-32.

13. Hutton JT, Morris JL. Long-acting carbidopa-levodopa in the management of moderate and advanced Parkinson's disease. Neurology 1992;42:51-56.

14. Rodnitzky R. The use of Sinemet CR in the management of mild to moderate Parkinson's disease. Neurology 1992;42 (suppl 1):44-50.

15. Block G, Liss C, Reines S, Irr J, Nibbelink D, The CR First Study Group. Comparison of immediate-release and controlled release carbidopa/levodopa in Parkinson's disease. A multicenter 5-year study. Eur Neurol 1997;37:23-27.

16. Lees AJ. Madopar HBS (hydrodynamically balanced system) in the treatment of Parkinson's disease. In: Korczyn AD, Melamed E, Youdim MBH eds. Advances in Neurology New York: Raven Press, 1990:475-82.

17. Koller W. Pharmacologic treatment of parkinsonian tremor. Arch Neurol 1986;43:126-127.

18. Jenner P. The rationale for the use of dopamine agonists in Parkinson's disease. Neurology 1995;45:S6-12.

19. Lees AJ, Stern GM. Sustained bromocriptine therapy in previously untreated patients with Parkinson's disease. J Neurol Neurosurg Psychiatry 1981;44:1020-1023.

20. Rascol O on behalf of the Study Group. A double-blind L-dopa controlled study of ropinirole in de novo patients with Parkinson's disease. Movement Disorders 1996;11 (Suppl 1):139.

21. Montastruc, JL, Rascol O, Senard JM. Current status of dopamine agonists in Parkinson's disease management. Drugs 1993;46:384-393

22. Hoehn MM, Elton RC. Low dosages of bromocriptine added to levodopa in Parkinson's disease. Neurology 1985;35:199-206.

23. Langtry J, Clissold SP. Pergolide: a review of its pharmacological properties and therapeutic potential in Parkinson's disease. Drugs 1990;39:491-506.

24. Olanow CW, Fahn S, Muenter M. A multicenter double-blind placebo-controlled trial of pergolide as an adjunct to Sinemet in Parkinson's disease. Movement Disorders 1994;9:40-47.

25. Thalamus C, Rayet S, Brefel C, Eagle S, Lopez-Gil K et al. Effect of food on the pharmacokinetics of ropinirole in patients with Parkinson's disease. Movement Disorders 1996;11 (Suppl 1):138.

26. Kreider M, Knox S, Gardiner D, Wheadon D. A multicenter double-blind study of ropinirole as an adjunct to L-dopa in Parkinson's disease. Neurology 1996;46 (Suppl):A475.

27. Wheadon DE, Wilson-Lynch K, Gardiner D, Kreider MS. Ropinirole, a non-ergoline D2 agonist, is effective in early parkinsonian patients not treated with L-dopa. Movement Disorders 1996;11(Suppl 1):162.

28. On behalf on the ropinirole 053 study group. To compare the efficacy at six months of ropinirole vs bromocriptine as early therapy in Parkinsonian patients. Movement Disorders 1996;11(Suppl 1):188.

29. Carvey PM. The case for neuroprotection with dopamine (DA) agonists. Movement Disorders 1996;11(Suppl 1):265.

30. Shannon KM. New alternatives for the management of early Parkinson's disease (PD). Movement Disorders 1996;11(Suppl 1):266.

31. Lieberman A for the Pramipexole Advanced Parkinson's Disease Study Group. Efficacy and safety of pramipexole in advanced Parkinson's disease patients with the "wearing-off" phenomenon. Neurology 1996;46(Suppl):A475.

32. Lera G, Vaamonde J, Rodriguez M, Obeso JA. A new long acting D-2 agonist for Parkinson's disease. Movement Disorders 1990:5(Suppl 1):78.

33. Pontiroli AE. Inhibition of basal and metoclopramide-induced prolactin release by cabergoline, an extremely long-acting dopaminergic drug. J Clin Endocrinol Metab 1987;65:1057-1059.

34. Ferrari C, Barbieri C, Caldara R, et al. Long-lasting prolactin lowering effect of cabergoline, a new dopamine agonist, in hyperprolactinemic patients. J Clin Endocrinol Met 1986;63:941-945.

35. Ahlskog JE, Muenter MD, Maraganore DM, Matsumoto JY, Lieberman A. Fluctuating Parkinson's disease. Arch Neurol 1994;51:1236-1241.

36. Hutton JT, Morris JL, Brewer MA. Controlled study of the antiparkinsonian activity and tolerability of cabergoline. Neurology 1993;43:613-616.

37. Gopinathan G, Teravainen H, Dambrosia JM. Lisuride in parkinsonism. Neurology 1981;31:371-376.

38. Obeso JA, Luquin MR, Martinez J. Intravenous lisuride corrects oscillations of motor performance in Parkinson's disease. Ann Neurol 1986;19:31-35.

39. Obeso JA, Luquin MR, Vaamonde J, et al. Subcutaneous administration of lisuride in the treatment of complex motor fluctuations in Parkinson's disease. J Neurol Trans 1988;27:S17-25.

40. Barker R, Duncan J, Lees AJ. Subcutaneous apomorphine as a diagnostic test for dopaminergic responsiveness in parkinsonian syndromes. Lancet 1989;1:675.

41. Gylys JA, Wright RN, Nicolosi WD, Buyinski JP, Crenshaw RR. BMY-25801, an antiemetic agent free of D2-dopamine receptor antagonist properties. J Pharmacol Exp Ther 1988;244:830-7.

42. Goiny M, Unvan-Moberg K. Effects of dopamine receptor antagonists on gastrin and vomiting responses to apomorphine. Naunyn-Schmiedeberg's Arch Pharmacol 1987;336:16-19.

43. Felten DL, Felten SY, Fuller RW et al. Chronic dietary pergolide preserves nigrostriatal neuronal integrity in aged-Fischer-344 rats. Neurobiol of Aging 1992;13:339-351.

44. Pearce RKB, Banerji T, Jenner P, Marsden CD. Effects of repeated treatment with L-dopa, bromocriptine and ropinirole in drug naive MPTP-treated common marmosets. British J Pharmacology;118:37P.

45. Rinne UK. Early combination of bromocriptine and levodopa in treatment of Parkinson's disease: a 5-year follow up. Neurology 1987;37:826-828

46. Montastruc JL, Rascol O, Senard JM, Rascol A. A randomised controlled study comparing bromocriptine to which levodopa was later added, with levodopa alone in previously untreated patients with Parkinson's disease: a five year follow up. Jour Neurol Neurosurg Psych 1994;57:1034-1038

47. Hely MA, Morris JGL, Reid WGJ, O'Sullivan DJ, Williamson PM. The Sydney Multicentre Study of Parkinson's Disease: a randomized, prospective five year study comparing low-dose bromocriptine with low dose levodopa-carbidopa. Jour Neurol Neurosurg Psych 1994;57:903-910.

48. Rinne UK. Early dopamine agonist therapy in Parkinson's disease. Movement Disorders 1989;4:S86-94.

49. Knoll J, Ecseri Z, Kelemen K, Nievel J, and Knoll B. Phenylisopropylmethylpropinylamine (E-250), a new spectrum psychic energizer. Arch INT Pharmacodyn 1965;155:154-164.

50. Elsworth JD, Glover V, Reynolds GP, et al. Deprenyl administration in man; a selective monoamine oxidase B inhibitor without the 'cheese effect'. Psychopharmacology 1978;57:33-38.

51. Golbe LI. Long-term efficacy and safety of deprenyl in advanced Parkinson's disease. Neurology 1989;39:1109-1111.

52. Birkmayer W, Riederer P, Youdim MBH et al. The potentiation of the anti-akinetic effect after L-dopa treatment by an inhibitor of MAO-B, Deprenil. J Neural Transm 1975;36:303-326.

53. Bodner RA, Lynch T, Lewis L, Kahn D. Serotonin syndrome. Neurology 1995;45:219-23.

54. Waters, C. Fluoxetine and selegiline-lack of significant interaction. Canadian Journal of Neurological Sciences 1994;21:259-261.

55. Parkinson Study Group. Effects of tocopherol and deprenyl on the progression of disability in early Parkinson's disease. N Engl J Med 1993;328:176-183.

56. Heikila RE, Manzino L, Cabbat FS, et al. Protection against the dopaminergic neurotoxicity of 1-methyl-4-phenyl-1,2,5,6-tetrahydropyridine by monoamine oxidase inhibitors. Nature 1984;311:467-469.

57. Birkmayer W, Knoll J, Riederer P. Increased life expectancy resulting from the addition of L-deprenyl to madopar treatment in Parkinson's disease; a long term study. J Neurol Trans 1985;64:113-27.

58. Olanow CW, Hauser RA, Gauger L et al. The effect of deprenyl and levodopa on the progression of Parkinson's disease. Ann Neurol 1995;38:771-777.

59. Tatton WG, Greenwood CE. Rescue of dying neurons: a new action for deprenyl in MPTP parkinsonism. Jour Neurosci Res 1991;30:666-72.

60. Tatton WG, Ju WY, Holland DP, Tai C, Kwan M. (-)-Deprenyl reduces PC12 cell apoptosis by inducing new protein synthesis. J Neurochem 1994;63:1572

61. Tatton WG, Chalmers-Redmond RME. Modulation of gene expression rather than monoamine oxidase inhibition: (-)-deprenyl-related compounds in controlling neurodegeneration. Neurology 1996;47(Suppl 3):S171-183.

62. Olanow CW. Selegiline: current perspectives on issues related to neuroprotection and mortality. Neurology 1996;47(Suppl 3):S210-216.

63. Lees AJ on behalf of the Parkinson's Disease Research Group of the United Kingdom. Comparison of therapeutic effects and mortality data of levodopa and levodopa combined with selegiline in patients with early, mild Parkinson's disease. BJM 1995;1602-1607.

64. Maki-Ikola O, Kilkku O, Heinonen E. Effect of adding selegiline to levodopa in early, mild Parkinson's disease: other studies have not shown increased mortality [letter]. BMJ 1996;312:702-703.

65. Axelrod J, Senoh S, Witkop B. O-methylation of catechol amines in vivo. J Biol Chem 1958;233:697-701.

66. Guldberg HC, Marsden CA. Catechol-O-methyl transferase: pharmacological aspects and physiological role. Pharmacol Rev 1975;27:135-206.

67. Nissenen E, Tuominen R, Perhoniemi V, Kaakkola S. Catechol-O-methyltransferase activity in human and rat small intestine. Life Sci 1988;42:2609-2614.

68. Kastner A, Anglade P, Bounaix C, Damier P, Javoy-Agid F et al. Immunohistochemical study of catechol-O-methyltransferase in the human mesostriatal system. Neuroscience 1994;62:449-457.

69. Reeches A, Meilke LR, Fahn S. 3-O-methyldopa inhibits rotations induced by levodopa in rats after unilateral destruction of the nigrostriatal pathway. Neurology 1982;32:887-888.

70. Nutt JG, Woodward WR, Gancher ST, Merrick D. 3-O-methyldopa and the response to levodopa in Parkinson's disease. Ann Neurol 1987;21:584-588.

71. Kaakkola S, Wurtman RJ. Effects of catechol-O-methyltransferase inhibitors and L-3, 4-dihydroxyphenylalanine with or without carbidopa on extracellular dopamine in rat striatum. J Neurochem 1993;60:137-144.

72. Dingemanse J, Jorga K, Zurcher G, Schmitt M, Sedek G et al. Pharmokinetic-pharmacodynamic interaction between the COMT inhibitor tolcapone and single-dose levodopa. Br J Clin Pharmacol 1995;40:253-262.

73. Goetz CG. Influence of COMT inhibition on levodopa therapy. Movement Disorders 1996;11(Suppl 1):271.

74. Waters CH, Kurth MC, Shulman L, Bailey P, Shale H et al. Evaluation of the efficacy and safety of Tolcapone (Tasmar) in Parkinson's Disease patients with a stable response to levodopa. Neurology 1996;46(Suppl):A160.

75. Dorflinger EE, Rajput A, Martin W, Saint-Hilaire MH, Chernik D et al. Multicenter evaluation of Tolcapone (Tasmar) when given together with levodopa to Parkinson's disease patients who exhibit end-of-dose wearing off. Neurology 1996;46(Suppl):A474.

76. Kaakkola S, Teravainen H, Ahtila S, Rita H, Gordin A. Effect of entacapone, a COMT inhibitor, on clinical disability and levodopa metabolism in parkinsonism patients. Neurology 1994;44:77-80.

77. Keranen T, Gordin A, Harjola VP, Karlsson M, Lorpela K. The effect of catechol-O-methyl transferase inhibition by entacapone on the pharmacokinetics and metabolism of levodopa in healthy volunteers. Clin Neuropharm 1993;16:145-156.

78. Kieburtz K for the Parkinson Study Group. The COMT inhibitor entacapone improves parkinsonian features in fluctuating patients. Movement Disorders 1996;11(Suppl 1):268.

79. Jabbari B, Scherokman B, Gunderson CH et al. Treatment of movement disorders with trihexyphenidyl. Movement Disorders 19889;4:202-212.

80. Butzer JF, Silver DE, Sahs AL. Amantadine in Parkinson's disease: a double-blind placebo-controlled cross-over study with long-term follow-up. Neurology 1975;25:603-606.

81. Gerlak RP, Clark R, Stump JM et al. Amantadine-dopamine interaction. Science 1970;169:203-204.

Chapter 6 references

1. Fahn S. "On-off" phenomenon with levodopa therapy in parkinsonism.
Clinical and pharmacologic correlates and the effect of intramuscular pyridoxine.
Neurology 1974;24:431-441.

2. Marsden CD, Parkes JD. "On-off" effects in patients with Parkinson's disease on chronic levodopa therapy. Lancet 1976;1:292-296.

3. Sage JI, Mark M. The rationale for continuous dopaminergic stimulation in patients with Parkinson's disease (review). Neurology 1992;42:S23-8

4. Chase TN, Mouradian MM, Engber TM. Motor response complications and the function of striatal efferent systems. Neurology 1993;43:S23-27.

5. Muenter MD, Sharpless NS, Tyce GM, Darly FL. Patterns of dystonia ("I-D-I" and "D-I-D") in response to L-dopa therapy for Parkinson's disease. Mayo Clin Proc 1977;52:163-174.

6. Mones RJ, Elizan TS, Siegel GJ. Analysis of L-dopa induced dyskinesias in 51 patients with parkinsonism. J Neurol Neurosurg Psychiatry 1971;34:668-73.

7. McHale DM, Sage JI, Sonsalla PK, Vitagliano D. Complex dystonia of Parkinson's disease: clinical features and relation to plasma levodopa profile. Clinical Neuropharmacology 1990;13:164-170.

8. Poewe WH, Lees AJ, Stern GM. Low-dose L-dopa therapy in Parkinson's disease; a 6-year follow up. Neurology 1986;36:1528-1530.

9. Hauser RA, Zesiewicz TA, Factor SA, Guttman M, Weiner W. Clinical trials of add-on medications in Parkinson's disease: efficacy versus usefulness. Parkinsonism and related disorders, 1997; 3:1-6.

10. Giladi N, McMahon D, Przedborski S, Flaster E, Guillory S, Kostic V, Fahn S. Motor blocks in Parkinson's disease. Neurology 1992;42:333-9.

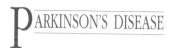

Chapter 7 references

1. Pearce RKB, Banerji T, Jenner P, Marsden CD. Effects of repeated treatment with L-dopa, bromocriptine and ropinirole in drug naive MPTP-treated common marmosets. British J Pharmacology;118:37P.

2. Montastruc JL, Rascol O, Senard JM, Rascol A. A randomised controlled study comparing bromocriptine to which levodopa was later added, with levodopa alone in previously untreated patients with Parkinson's disease: a five year follow up. J Neurol, Neurosurg, and Psych 1994;57:1034-1038.

3. Hely MA, Morris JGL, Reid WGJ, O'Sullivan DJ, Williamson PM. The Sydney Multicentre Study of Parkinson's disease: a randomized, prospective five year study comparing low dose bromocriptine with low dose levodopa-carbidopa. J Neurol Neurosurg Psych 1994;57:903-910.

4. Block G, Liss C, Reines S, Irr J, Nibbelink D, The CR First Study Group. Comparison of immediate-release and controlled release carbidopa/levodopa in Parkinson's disease. A multicenter 5-year study. Eur Neurol 1997;37:23-27.

5. Carter JH, Nutt JG, Woodward WR, Hatcher LF, Trotman TL. Amount and distribution of dietary protein affects clinical response to levodopa in Parkinson's disease. Neurology 1989;39:552-556.

6. Kurth MC, Tetrud JW, Irwin I, Lynes WH, Langston JW. Oral levodopa/carbidopa solution versus tablets in Parkinson's disease patients with severe fluctuations: a pilot study. Neurology 1993;43:1036-1039.

7. Lieberman A, Dziatolowski M, Kupersmith M, Serby M, Goodgold A, Korein J, Goldstein M. Dementia in Parkinson's disease. Ann Neurol 1979;6:355-359.

8. Baldessarini RJ, Frankenburg FR. Drug therapy: clozapine-a novel antipsychotic agent. N Engl J Med 1991;324:746-756.

References Chapter 8

1. Cummings JL. Depression and Parkinson's disease: a review. Am J Psychiatry 1992;149:443-454.

2. Ehmann TS, Beninger RJ, Gawal MJ, Riopelle RJ. Depressive symptoms in Parkinson's disease: a comparison with disabled control subjects. J Geriatr Psychiatry Neurol 1990;2:3-9.

3. Starkstein SE, Preziosi TJ, Bolduc PL, Robinson RG. Depression in Parkinson's disease. J Nerv Ment Dis 1990;178:27-31.

4. Gotham AM, Brown RG, Marsden CD. Depression in Parkinson's disease: a quantitative and qualitative analysis. J Neurol Neurosurg Psychiatry 1986;49:381-389.

5. Celesia GC, Wanamaker WM. Psychiatric disturbances in Parkinson's disease. Dis Nerv Syst 1972;33:577-583.

6. Mayeux R, Stern Y, Williams JBW, Cote L, Frantz A, Dyrenfurth I. Clinical and biochemical features of depression in Parkinson's disease. Am J Psychiatry 1986;143:756-759.

7. Mayeux R, Stern Y, Sano M, Williams JB, Cote LJ. The relationship of serotonin to depression in Parkinson's disease. Mov Disord 1988;3:237-244.

8. Andersen J, Aabro E, Gulmann N, Hjelmsted A, Pedersen HE. Anti-depressive treatment in Parkinson's disease: a controlled trial of the effect of nortriptyline in patients with Parkinson's disease treated with L-dopa. Acta Neurol Scan 1980;52:210-219.

9. Laitenen L. Desipramine in treatment of Parkinson's disease. Acta Neurol Scand 1969;45:109-113.

10. Goetz CG, Tanner CM, Klawans HL. Bupropion in Parkinson's disease. Neurology 1984;34:1092-1094.

11. Jansen-Steur ENH. Increase of Parkinson disability after fluoxetine medication. Neurology 1993;43:211-213.

12. Jimenez-Jimenez FJ, Tejeiro J, Martinez-Junquera G, Cabrera-Valdivia F, Alarcon J, et al. Parkinsonism exacerbated by paroxetine. Neurology 1994;44:2406.

13. Hauser RA, Zesiewicz TA. Sertraline for the treatment of depression in Parkinson's disease. Movement Disorders (In Press).

14. Sternbach H. The serotonin syndrome. Am J Psychiatry 1991;148:705-713.

15. Nirenberg DW, Semprebon M. The central nervous system serotonin syndrome. Clin Pharmacol Ther 1993;84-88.

16. Tackley RM, Tregaskis B. Fatal disseminated intravascular coagulation following a monoamine oxidase inhibitor/tricyclic interaction. Anaesthesia 1987;42:760-763.

17. Corkeron MA. Serotonin syndrome - a potentially fatal complication of antidepressant therapy. Med J Austral 1995;163:481-482.

18. Waters CH. Fluoxetine and selegiline - lack of significant interaction. Can J Neurol 1994;21:259-261.

19. Hickler RB, Thompson GR, Fox LM, Hamlin JT. Successful treatment of orthostatic hypotension with 9-alpha-fluorohydrocortisone. N Engl J Med 1959;261:788-791.

20. Kaufman H, Brannan T, Krakoff L, Yahr MD, Mandeli J. Treatment of orthostatic hypotension due to autonomic failure with a peripheral alpha-adrenergic agonist (midodrine). Neurology 1988;38:951-956.

21. Davies B, Bannister R, Sever P. Pressor amines and monoamineoxidase inhibitors for treatment of postural hypotension in autonomic failure: limitations and hazards. Lancet 1978;1:172-175.

22. McTavish D, Goa KL. Midodrine: a review of its pharmacological properties and therapeutic use in orthostatic hypotension and secondary hypotensive disorders. Drugs 1989;38:757-777.

23. Pittner H, Stormann H, Enzenhofer R. Pharmacodynamic actions of midodrine, a new alpha-adrenergic stimulating agent, and its main metabolite, ST 1059. Arzneim Forsch 1976;26:2145-2154.

24. Zachariah PK, Bloedow DC, Moyer TP, Sheps SG, Schirger A, et al. Pharmacodynamics of midodrine, an antihypotensive agent. Clin Pharmacol Ther 1986;39:586-591.

25. Jankovic J, Gilden JL, Hiner BC, Kaufman H, Brown DC. Neurogenic orthostatic hypotension: a double-blind placebo-controlled study with midodrine.
Am J Med 1993;95:38-48.

26. Jost WH, Schimrigk K. Constipation in Parkinson's disease. Klinische Wochenschrift 1991;69:906-909.

27. Edwards LL, Quigley EMM, Harned RK, Hofman R, Pfeiffer R. Characterization of swallowing and defecation in Parkinson's disease. Am J Gastroenterol 1994;89:15-25.

28. Ashraf W, Pfeiffer R, Quigely EMM. Anorectal manometer in the assessment of anorectal function in Parkinson's disease: a comparison with chronic idiopathic constipation.
Movement Disorders 1994;9:655-663.

29. Mathers SE, Kempster PA, Law PJ, et al. Anal sphincter dysfunction in Parkinson's disease. Arch Neurol 1989;46:1061-1064.

30. Oyanagi K, Wakabayashi K, Ohama E, Takeda S, Horikawa Y, Morita T, Ikuta F. Lewy bodies in the lower sacral parasympathetic neurons of a patient with Parkinson's disease. Acta Neuropathol 1990;80:558-559.

31. Mathers SE, Kempster PA, Swash M, Lees AJ. Constipation and paradoxical puborectalis contraction in anismus and Parkinson's disease: a dystonic phenomenon?
J Neurol Neurosurg Psych 1988;51:1503-1507.

32. Koller WC, Silver DE, Lieberman A. An algorithm for the management of Parkinson's disease. Neurology 1994;44:S19-20.

33. Jost WH, Schimrigk K. The effect of cisapride on delayed colonic transit time in patients with idiopathic Parkinson's disease. Wiener Klinische Wochenschrift 1994;106:673-6.

34. Neira WD, Sanchea V, Mena MA, Yebenes JG. The effects of cisapride on plasma L-dopa levels and clinical response in Parkinson's disease. Movement Disorders 1995;10:66-70.

35. Edwards LL, Pfeiffer RF, Quigley EMM, Hofman R, Balluff M. Gastrointestinal symptoms in Parkinson's disease. Movement Disorders 1991;6:151-156.

36. Edwards LL, Quigley EMM, Pfeiffer RF. Gastrointestinal dysfunction in Parkinson's disease: frequency and pathophysiology. Neurology 1992;42:726-732.

37. Bird MR, Woodward MC, Gibson EM, Phyland DJ, Fonda D. Asymptomatic swallowing disorders in elderly patients with Parkinson's disease: a description of findings on clinical examination and videofluoroscopy in sixteen patients. Age and Ageing 1994;23:251-4.

38. Qualman SJ, Haupt HM, Yang P, Hamilton SR. Esophageal Lewy bodies associated with ganglion cell loss in achalasia. Similarity to Parkinson's disease.
Gastroenterology 1984;87:848-56.

39. Wang SJ, Chia LG, Hsu CY, Lin WY, Kao CH, Yeh SH. Dysphagia in Parkinson's disease. Assessment by solid phase radionuclide scintigraphy. Clin Nuc Med 1994;19:405-7.

40. Wintzen AR, Badrising UA, Roos RA, Vielvoye J, Liauw L, Pauwels EK. Dysphagia in ambulant patients with Parkinson's disease: common, not dangerous. Can J Neur Sci 1994;212:53-6.

41. Bushman M, Dobmeyer SM, Leeker L, Perlmutter JS. Swallowing abnormalities and their responses to treatment in Parkinson's disease. Neurology 1989;39:1309-1314.

42. Khan Z, Starer P, Bhola A. Urinary incontinence in female Parkinson's disease patients. Urology 1989;33:486-9.

43. Suchowersky O, Furtado S, Rohs G. Beneficial effect of intranasal desmopressin for nocturnal polyuria in Parkinson's disease. Movement Disorders 1995;10:337-40.

44. Lipe, H, Longstreth WT, Bird TD, Linde M. Sexual function in married men with Parkinson's disease compared to married men with arthritis. Neurology 1990;40:1347-1349.

45. Rosen RC, Kostis JB, Jekelis AW. Beta-blocker effects on sexual function in normal males. Arch Sex Behavior 1988;17:241-55.

46. Smith PJ, Talbert RL. Sexual dysfunction with antihypertensive and antipsychotic agents. Clinical Pharmacy 1986;5:373-84.

47. Bilowit DS. Establishing physical objectives in the rehabilitation of patients with Parkinson's disease (gymnasium activities). Phys Ther Rev 1956;36:176-178.

48. Hurwitz A. The benefit of a home exercise regimen for ambulatory Parkinson's disease patients. J Neurosci Nursing 1989;21:180-184.

49. Comella CL, Stebbins GT, Brown-Toms BA, Goetz C. Physical therapy and Parkinson's disease: a controlled clinical trial. Neurology 1994;44:376-378.

Chapter 9

1. Pollack LJ, Davis L. Muscle tone in Parkinsonian states. Arch Neurol Psych 1930;23:303-319.

2. Bucy PC. Cortical extirpation in the treatment of involuntary movements. Am J Surg 1948;75:257-263.

3. Putnam TJ. Treatment of unilateral paralysis agitans by section of the lateral pyramidal tract. Arch Neurol Psych 1940;44:950-976.

4. Walker AE. Cerebral pedunculotomy for the relief of involuntary movements. J Nerv Ment Dis 1952;116:766-775.

5. Cooper IS. Parkinsonism: Its Medical and Surgical Therapy. Springfield, Ill., Charles C. Thomas 1961.

6. Meyers R. The modification of alternating tremors, rigidity and festination by surgery of the basal ganglia. Res Publ Assoc Res Nerv Ment Dis 1942;21:602-665.

7. Meyers R. Surgical experiments in the therapy of certain "extrapyramidal" diseases: a current evaluation. Acta Psychiatrica et Neurologica 1951;Suppl 67:3.

8. Fenelon F. Essais de traitment neurochirurgical du syndrome parkinsonen par intervention direct sur les voies extrapyramidales immediatement sous-striopallidales (anse lenticulaire) Rev Neurol 1950;83:437-440.

9. Fenelon F, Theibant F. Resultats du traitement neurochirurgical d'une rigidite parkinsonienne par intervention striopallidale unilaterale. Rev Neurol 1950;83:280.

10. Guiot G, Brion S. Traitement des mouvements anormaux par la coagulation pallidale. Rev Neurol 1953;83:578-580.

11. Cooper IS. The Neurosurgical Alleviation of Parkinsonism. Springfield Ill., Charles C. Thomas, 1956.

12. Abbie AA. Morphology of fore-brain arteries, with especial reference to evolution of basal ganglia. J Anat 1934;68:433-470.

13. Spiegel EA, Wycis HT, Marks M, et al. Stereotaetic apparatus for operation on the human brain. Science 1947;106:349-350.

14. Spiegel EA, Wycis HT. Ansotomy in paralysis agitans. Arch Neurol Psych 1954;71:598-614.

15. Speigel EA, Wycis HT, Thur C. The stereoencephalotome. J Neurosurg 1951;8:452-453.

16. Hassler R, Reichert T. Indikationen and localizations: Methode der gezielten Hirnoperationen. Nevenarzt 1954;25:411-447.

17. Cooper IS, Bravo G. Chemopallidectomy and chemothalamectomy. J Neurosurg. 1958;15:244-250.

18. Selby G. Stereotactic surgery for the relief of Parkison's disease. Part I: A critical review. J Neurol Sci 1967;5:315-342.

19. Mundinger F, Riechert T. Esgelnisse der sterotaktischen Hirnoperationen bei extrapyramidalen Bewegungsstrorungen auf Grund postoperativer und Langzeituntersuchungen. Dtsch Z Nervenheilk 1961;182:542-576.

20. Krayenbuhl H, Yasargil MG. Ergebnisse der sterotaktischen Operationen beim Parkinsonismus, insbesondere der doppelseitgen Eingriffe. Dtsch Z Nervenheilk 1961;182:530-541.

21. Narabayashi H, Ikuma T, Shibiba S. Discussion of the speeches by Dr. Buch and Dr. Walker. Rapports and Discussions I, 1st Int Congress Neurol Sci, Brussels, 1957. Acta Medica Belgica. 1957:138-142.

22. Svennilson E, Torvik A, Lowe R, et al. Treatment of parkinsonism by stereotactic thermolesions in the pallidal region. Acta Psychiat Scand 1960;35:358-377.

23. Spiegel EA, Wycis HT. Stereoencephalotomy. Part 2. Clinical and Physiological Applications. New York, Grune and Stratton, 1962.

24. Tasker RR. Surgical aspects: symposium on extrapyramidal disease. Applied Therapeutics 1967;9:454-462.

25. Tasker RR, Siqueira J, Hawrylyshyn P, et al. What happened to VIM thalamotomy for Parkinson's disease? Appl Neurophysiol 1983;46:68-83.

26. Kelly PJ, Ahlskog JE, Goerss SJ, et al. Computer-assisted stererotactic ventralis lateralis thalamotomy with microelectrode recording control in patients with Parkinson's disease. Mayo Clin Proc 1987;62:655-664.

27. Kelly PH, Gillingham FJ. The long-term results of stereotactic surgery and L-dopa therapy in patients with Parkinson's disease. J Neurosurg 1980;53:332-337.

28. Matsumoto K, Schichijo F, Fukami T. Long-term follow-up review of cases of Parkinson's disease after unilateral or bilateral thalamotomy. J Neurosurg 1984;60:1033-1044.

29. Miyamoto T, Bekku H, Moriyama E, et al. Present role of sterotactic thalamotomy for parkinsonism. Retrospective analysis of operative results and thalamic lesions in computed tomograms. Appl Neurophysiol 1985;48:294-304.

30. Mundinger F. Postoperative and long-term results of 1,561 sterotactic operations in parkinsonism. Appl Neurophysiol 1985;48:293.

31. Narabayashi H, Maeda T, Yokochi F. Long-term follow-up study of nucleus ventralis intermedius and ventrolateralis thalamotomy using a microeletrode technique in parkinsonism. Appl Neurophysiol 1987;50:330-337.

32. Nagaseki Y, Shibazaki T, Hirai T, et al. Long-term follow-up results of selective VIM-thalamotomy. J Neurosurg 1986;65:296-302.

33. Scott RM, Brody JA, Cooper IS. The effect of thalamotomy on the progress of unilateral Parkinson's disease. J Neurosurg 1970;32:286-288.

34. Tasker RR. Thalamotomy. Neurology Clinics of North America 1990; 1:841-864.

35. Krayenbuhl H, Wyss OAM, Yasargil MG. Bilateral thalamotomy and pallidotomy as treatment for bilateral parkinsonism. J Neurosurg 1961;18:429-444.

36. Matsumoto K, Asano T, Baba T, et al. Long-term follow-up results of bilateral thalamotomy for parkinsonism. J Neurophysiol 1976;39:257-260.

37. Riechert T. Stereotactic brain operations: methods, clinical aspects, indications. Bern, Hans Huber 1980, pp. 213-304.

38. Fox MW, Ahlskog JE, Kelly PJ. Stereotactic ventrolateralis thalamotomy for medically refractory tremor in post-levodopa era Parkinson's disease patients. J Neurosurg 1991;75:723-730.

39. Diederich N, Goetz CG, Stebbins GT, et al. Blinded evaluation confirms long-term asymmetric effect of unilateral thalamotomy or subthalamotomy on tremor in Parkinson's disease. Neurology 1992;42:1311-1314.

40. Laitinen LV. Thalamic targets in stereotaetic treatment of Parkinson's disease. J Neurosurg 1966;24:82-85.

41. Cooper IS. Surgical treatment of parkinsonism. Ann Rev Med 1965;16:309-330.

42. Benabid AL, Pollak P, Louveau A, et al. Combined (thalamotomy and stimulation) stereotactic surgery of the VIM thalamic nucleus for bilateral Parkinson's disease. Appl Neurophysiol 1987;50:344-346.

43. Benabid AL, Pollak P, Gervason C, et al. Long-term suppression of tremor by chronic stimulation of the ventral intermediate thalamic nucleus. Lancet 1991;337:403-406.

44. Blond S, Siegfried J. Thalamic stimulation for the treatment of tremor and other movement disorders. Acta Neurochirurgica 1991;52:109-111.

45. Benabid AL, Pollak P, Gao D, et al. Chronic electrical stimulation of the ventralis intermedius nucleus of the thalamus as a treatment of movement disorders. J Neurosurg 1996;84:203-214.

46. Blond S, Caparros-Lefebvre D, Parker F, et al. Control of tremor and involuntary movement disorders by chronic stereotactic stimulation of the ventral intermediate thalamic nucleus. J Neurosurg 1992;77:62-68.

47. Laitinen LV, Bergenheim AT, Hariz MI. Leksell's posteroventral pallidotomy in the treatment of Parkinson's disease. J Neurosurg 1992;76:53-61.

48. Laitinen LV, Bergenheim AT, Hariz MI. Ventroposterolateral pallidotomy can abolish all parkinsonian symptoms. Stereotact Funct Neurosurg 1992;58:14-21.

49. Dogali M, Fazzini E, Kolodny E, Eidelberg D, Sterio D, Devinsky O, Beric A. Stereotactic ventral pallidotomy for Parkinson's disease. Neurology 1995;45:753-761.

50. Lang AE, Lozano A, Duff J, Miyasaki J, Galvez-Jiminez N, Hutchison W, Tasker R, Dostrovsky J. Posteroventral medial pallidotomy in Parkinson's disease. Movement Disorders 1995;10:4.

51. Baron MS, Vitek JL, Bakay RAE, et al. Treatment of advanced Parkinson's disease by posterior GPi pallidotomy: 1-year results of a pilot study. Ann Neurol 1996;40:355-366.

52. Siegfried J, Lippitz B. Bilateral chronic electrostimulation of ventroposterolateral pallidum: A new therapeutic approach for alleviating all parkinsonian symptoms. Neurosurgery 1994;35:1126-1130.

53. Limousin P, Pollak P, Benazzouz A, Hoffmann D, LeBas JF, Broussolle E, Perret JE, Benabid AL. Effect on parkinsonian signs and symptoms of bilateral subthalamic nucleus stimulation. Lancet 1995;345:91-95.

54. Perlow M, Freed WJ, Hoffer BJ, et al. Brain grafts reduce motor abnormalities produced by destruction of nigro-striatal dopamine system. Science 1979;204:643-647.

55. Bjorklund A, Kromer LF, Stenevi U. Cholinergic reinnervation of the rat hippocampus by septal implants is stimulated by perforant path lesion. Brain Res 1979;173:57-64.

56. Bjorklund A, Stenevi U, Schmidt RH, et al. Intracerebral grafting of neuronal cell suspensions. I. Introduction and general methods of preparation. Acta Physiol Scand 1983;522:9-18.

57. Mahalick TJ, Finger TE, Stromberg I, et al. Substantia nigra transplants into denervated striatum of the rat: Ultrastructure of graft-host interconnections. J Comp Neurol 1985;240:60-70.

58. Wuerthele SM, Freed WJ, Olson L, et al. Effects of dopamine agonists and antagonists on the electrical activity of substantia nigra neurons tranplanted into the lateral ventricle of the rat. Exp Brain Res 1981;44:1-10.

59. Schmidt RH, Ingvar M, Lindvall O, et al. Functional activity of substantia nigra grafts reinnervating the striatum: neurotransmitter metabolism and [14C]-2deoxy-D-glucose autoradiography. J Neurochem 1982;38:737-748.

60. Brundin P, Bjorklund A. Survival, growth and function of dopaminergic neurons grafted to the brain. Prog Brain Res 1987;71:293-308.

61. Sladek JR, Collier TC, Haber SN, et al. Survival and growth of fetal catecholamine neurons transplanted into the primate brain. Brain Res Bull 1986;17:809-818.

62. Bakay RAE, Barrow DL, Fiandca MS, et al. Biochemical and behavioral correction of MPTP-like syndrome by fetal transplantation. Ann NY Acad Sci 1987;495:623-640.

63. Sladek JR, Redmond DE, Collier TC, et al. Fetal dopamine neural grafts: extended reversal of methylphenyltetrahydropyridine-induced parkinsonism in primates. Prog Brain Res 1988;78:497-506.

64. Fine A, Hunt SB, Oertel WH, et al. Transplantation of embryonic dopaminergic neurons to the corpus striatum of marmosets rendered parkinsonian by 1-methyl-4-phenyl-1,2,3,6-tetrahydropyridine. Prog Brain Res 1988;78:479-490.

65. Bohn MC, Cupit L, Marciano F, et al. Adrenal medulla autografts into the basal ganglia of cebus monkeys: injury-induced regeneration. Exp Neurol 1988;102:76-91.

66. Backlund EO, Granberg PO, Hamerger B, et al. Transplantation of adrenal medullary tissue to striatum in parkinsonism. First clinical trials. J Neurosurg 1985;62:169-173.

67. Lindvall O, Backlund EO, Farde L, et al. Transplantation in Parkinson's disease: two cases of adrenal medullary grafts to the putamen. Ann Neurol 1987;22:457-468.

68. Madrazo I, Drucker-Colin R, Diaz V, et al. Open microsurgical autograft of adrenal medulla to right caudate nucleus in two patients with intractable Parkinson's disease. NEJM 1987;316:831-834.

69. Lieberman A, Ransohoff J, Berczeller P, et al. Neural and adrenal medullary transplants as a treatment for Parkinson's disease and other neurodegenerative disorders. Trends Clin Neurol 1988;4:1-15.

70. Penn RD, Goetz CG, Tanner CM, et al. The adrenal medullary transplant operation for Parkinson's disease: clinical observations in five patients. Neurosurgery 1988;22:999-1004.

71. Allen GS, Burns RS, Tulipan NB, et al. Adrenal medullary transplantation to the caudate nucleus in Parkinson's disease. Initial clinical results in 18 patients. Arch Neurol 1989; 46:487-491.

72. Goetz CG, Olanow CW, Koller WC, et al. Multicenter study of autologous adrenal medullary transplantation to the corpus striatum in patients with advanced Parkinson's disease. NEJM 1989;320:337-341.

73. Jankovic J. Grossman R, Goodman C, et al. Clinical, biochemical, and neuropathologic findings following transplantation of adrenal medulla to the caudate nucleus for treatment of Parkinson's disease. Neurology 1989;39:1227-1234.

74. Kelly PJ, Ahlskog JE, vanHeerden JA, et al. Adrenal medullary autograft transplantation into the striatum of patients with Parkinson's disease. Mayo Clin Proc 1989;64:282-290.

75. Ahlskog JE, Kelly PH, vanHeerden JA, et al. Adrenal medullary transplantation into the brain for treatment of Parkinson's disease: clinical outcome and neurochemical studies. Mayo Clin Proc 1990;65:305-328.

76. Apuzzo MLJ, Neal JH, Waters CH, et al. Utilization of unilateral and bilateral stereotactically placed adrenomedullary-striatal autografts in parkinsonian humans: rationale, techniques and observations. Neurosurgery 1990;26:746-757.

77. Koller WC, Waxman M, Morantz R. Adrenal neural transplants in Parkinson's disease. Adv Neurol 1990;53:559-565.

78. Olanow CW, Koller WC, Goetz CG, et al. Autologous transplantation of adrenal medulla in Parkinson's disease. Arch Neurol 1990;47:1286-1289.

79. Goetz CG, Stebbins GT, Klawans HL, et al. United Parkinson Foundation neurotransplantation registry on adrenal medullary transplant: presurgical, and 1-and 2-year follow-up. Neurology 1991;41:1719-1722.

80. Frank F, Sturiale C, Gaist C, et al. Adrenal medulla autograft in a human brain for Parkinson's disease. Acta Neurochir 1988;94:39.

81. Hurtig H, Joyce J, Sladek JR, et al. Post-mortem analysis of adrenal medulla-to-caudate autogaft in a patient with Parkinson's disease. Ann Neurol 1989;25:607-614.

82. Waters C, Itabashi HH, Apuzzo MLJ, et al. Adrenal to caudate transplantation - post mortem study. Mov Disord 1990;5:248-250.

83. Kordower JH, Cochran E, Penn R, et al. Putative chromaffin cell survival and enhanced host derived TH-fiber innervation following a functional adrenal medulla autogaft for Parkinson's disease. Ann Neurol 1991;29:405-412.

84. Hirsch EC, Duyckaerts C, Javoy-Agid F, et al. Does adrenal graft enhance recovery of dopaminergic neurons in Parkinson's disease? Ann Neurol 1990;27:676-682.

85. Freeman TB, Spence MS, Boss BD, et al. Development of dopaminergic neurons in the human substantia nigra. Exp Neurol 1991;113:344-353.

86. Verney C, Zecevic N, Nikolic B, et al. Early evidence of catecholaminergic cell groups in 5-and 6-week -old human embryos using tyrosine hydroxylase and dopamine-B-hydroxylase immunocytochemistry. Neuroscience Letters 1991;131:121.

87. Lindvall O, Rechncrona S, Gustaavii N, et al. Fetal dopamine-rich mesencephalic grafts in Parkinson's disease. Lancet 1988;1483-1484.

88. Lindvall O, Rehncrona S, Brundin P, et al. Human fetal dopamine neurons grafted into the striatum in two patients with Parkinson's disease: a detailed account of methodology and 6 month follow-up. Arch Neurol 1989;46:615-631.

89. Lindvall O, Brundin P, Widner H, et al. Grafts of fetal dopamine neurons survive and improve motor function in Parkinson's disease. Science 1990;247:574-577.

90. Lindvall O, Widner H, Rehncrona S, et al. Transplantation of fetal dopamine neurons in Parkinson's disease: one-year clinical and neurophysiological observations in two patients with putaminal implants. Ann Neurol 1992;31:155-165.

91. Sawle GV, Bloomfield PM, Bjorklund A, et al. Transplantation of fetal dopamine neurons in Parkinson's disease: PET 18F-6- fluorodopa studies in two patients with putaminal implants. Ann Neurol 1992;31:166-173.

92. Freed CR, Breeze RE, Rosenberg NL, et al. Transplantation of human fetal dopamine cells for Parkinson's disease. Results at one year. Arch Neurol 1990;47:505-512.

93. Freed CR, Breeeze RE, Rosenberg NL, et al. Survival of implanted fetal dopamine cells and neurologic improvement 12 to 46 months after transplantation for Parkinson's disease. NEJM 1992;327:1549-1555.

94. Spencer DD, Robbins RJ, Naftolin F, et al. Unilateral transplantation of human fetal mesencephalic tissue into the caudate nucleus of patients with Parkinson's disease. NEJM 1992;327:1541-1548.

95. Widner H, Tetrud J, Rehncrona S, et al. Bilateral fetal mesencephalic grafting in two patients with parkinsonism induced by 1-methyl-4-phenyl-1,2,3,6-tetrahydropyridine (MPTP). NEJM 1992;327:1556-63.

96. Freeman TB, Olanow CW, Hauser RA, Nauert GM, Smith DA, Borlongan CV, Sanberg PR, Holt Da, Kordower JH, Vingerhoets JG, Snow BJ, Calne D, Gauger LL. Bilateral fetal nigral transplantation into the postcommissural putamen in Parkinson's disease. Ann Neurol 1995;38:379-388.

97. Kordower JH, Freeman TB, Snow BA, Vingerhoets FJG, Mufson EJ, Sanberg PR, Hauser RA, Smith DA, Nauert GM, Perl DP, Olanow CW. Neuropathological evidence of graft survival and striatal reinnervation after the transplantation of fetal mesencephalic tissue in a patient with Parkinson's disease. NEJM 1995;332:1118-1124.

INDEX

ACKNOWLEDGMENTS

Figure 1-1. *Reprinted with kind permission from Duvoisin RC, Sage J. Parkinson's Disease: A Guide for Patient and Family. 4th Edition. Lippincot-Raven, 1996.*

Figure 1-2. *Reprinted with kind permission from Jankovic J, Tolosa E, Eds. Parkinson's Disease and Movement Disorders. Williams and Wilkins, 1993.*

Figure 1-5. *Reprinted with kind permission from Calne DB. Parkinsonism: Physiology, Pharmacology and Treatment. Edward Arnold, 1970.*

Figure 1-7. *Reprinted with kind permission from Calne DB. New England Journal of Medicine 1993;329:1022.*

Figure 1-8. *Reprinted with kind permission from Calne DB. New England Journal of Medicine 1993;329:1023.*

Figure 1-9. *Reprinted with kind permission from Calne DB. New England Journal of Medicine 1993;329:1023.*

Figure 4-2. *Reprinted with kind permission from Olanow CW. Ann Neurol 1992;32:S3.*

Figure 4-3. *Reprinted with kind permission from Olanow CW. Ann Neurol 1992;32:S3.*

Figure 4-4. *Reprinted with kind permission from Olanow CW. Ann Neurol 1992;32:S3.*

Figure 4-5. *Reprinted with kind permission from Cedarbaum JM, Grancher ST. Neurologic Clinics 1992;10:544.*

Figure 4-6. *Reprinted with kind permission from DiMonte D. Neurology 1991;41:39.*

Figure 5-3. *Reprinted with kind permission from Appel SH, Ed. Current Neurology 1992;12:130.*

Figure 5-4. *Reprinted with kind permission from The Parkinson Study Group. New England Journal of Medicine 1993;328:178.*

Figure 5-5. *Reprinted with kind permission from Kaakkola S. Rinne UK, Gordin A. COMT Inhibition with Entacapone: a New Principle of Levodopa Extension. Koteva Oy, Tahitorni Oy; Finland 1996:13.*

Figure 5-6. *Reprinted with kind permission from Kaakkola S. Rinne UK, Gordin A. COMT Inhibition with Entacapone: a New Principle of Levodopa Extension. Koteva Oy, Tahitorni Oy; Finland 1996:14.*

Figure 5-7. *Reprinted with kind permission from Gordin A, Rinne UK. Rinne UK, Gordin A. COMT Inhibition with Entacapone: a New Principle of Levodopa Extension. Koteva Oy, Tahitorni Oy; Finland 1996:27.*